...The heart monitor slowed and stopped. *There was a moment of unreality, of vacantness, of not being anywhere. And then just as suddenly, the realization hit, and both my world and my body came crashing to the floor. I was helped to my feet and back to reality. Through my tears I could see my wife, or the person who used to be my wife, lying motionless. She looked uncomfortable, not peaceful. Aren't people supposed to look peaceful once they have been released from their battle with the illness? Who am I going to take advice from now? Who is going to teach me? Who can I hug? What was it like for her? The answers are not obvious.*

She was thirty-nine and I was forty-two. This was not supposed to happen. It was a bad day. Funeral arrangements were followed by a drive home to tell my children that their mother had died. The tears made the drive dangerous, raising other concerns. Let's not cause the children to lose both parents today...

...Kathy and Gary met on December 18, 1992. Fluorescents illuminated the room, encouraging blinding reality. He couldn't cry because it had been over two years since his wife died, and he had to present a picture of having "weathered the storm." Kathy couldn't cry because she was ill at ease among the widow veterans. But when they met, they did not need to cry or even speak. The hurt was communicated clearly, the need was mutually felt, the loneliness, emptiness, need and anger was all there in a glance. Introductions seemed redundant, but having done so, the basis for a life-long friendship, and more, had been established. Friends, relatives and support people all figure into the recovery from loss and grief, but this was something else.

We were young widows and widowers, a strange breed combining the end of a life with the strong life force of a living young person with so much potential. The task would be to harness that energy and pull it from the grip of the tragedy. This cannot be done alone. With our companions dead, could we allow ourselves to be open to this?

LOSS and FOUND

How we survived the loss of a young spouse

by

Kathy and Gary Young

calabash press

LOSS AND FOUND
How we survived the loss of a young spouse

Calabash Press

PRINTING HISTORY
Calabash edition / January 2002

ISBN: 0-9715092-0-4
lccn: 2001096775

Calabash Press
P.O. Box 8728, Calabasas, California 91372-8728
www.LossAndFound.com

PRINTED IN THE UNITED STATES OF AMERICA
10 9 8 7 6 5 4 3 2 1

**Publisher's Catalolging-in-Publication
(Provided by Quality Books, Inc.)**

Young, Gary, 1945-
    Loss and found : how we survived the loss of a young
spouse / by Gary and Kathy Young.
        p. cm.
    LCCN 2001096775
    ISBN 0-9715092-0-4

    1. Grief. 2. Bereavement--Psychological aspects.
3. Loss (Psychology) 4. Spouses--Death--Psychological
aspects.   I. Young, Kathy, 1952- II. Title.

To Kathie and Sandy

ACKNOWLEDGEMENTS

The insights and information contained within this book would be impossible without the help and encouragement of many young widows and widowers, support group leaders, most especially at Our House in Los Angeles and Kaiser Permanente in Panorama City, and psychologists .

We want to thank Jo-Ann Lautmann, Linda Cunningham, the many support leaders, and the young widows and widowers for their candor and openness when talking to us. Also, we want to thank the many support leaders, psycholgists, and widows that we have spoken to through our website and through the production of Gary's play, *Interruptions,* which played during summer of 2000 in Hollywood, with more to come.

We especially want to thank George and Bette Baulch, Robert and Beverly Natelson, and Rick Natelson for their continuing unconditional love and support.

Our experiences were personal, even though most moments are shared with the collective young widow/widower population. Everyone is different, of course, but our goal is to show how we handled our own young widowhood.

Some names, occupations and/or physical descriptions found in this book have been fictionalized to protect privacy.

Table of contents

Part II: Kathy's Story

INTRODUCTION

TO START

We could start with the tears, with the expectations dashed or the changes in our lives, and leave it at that. We could dwell on all of the disruptive things that happened during the several years of illness and after, leading up to the "crash." We could dwell on the positive lessons learned about the value of time and human life, or the lesson learned as our spouses died in our arms.

This book is not about dying. It is really about surviving. Not necessarily making sense out of the tragic, capricious, unnerving events that bombard us, but making grief manageable, rather than letting it manage us.

NOT TO START

Our recollections will make sense, but it's hard to make sense out of this type of situation, or even life in general. Maybe we can at least be intelligible about what occurred and the aftermath.

OKAY, WE START

For a second let's start at the end. The end of a young life is a kick in the butt. A second kick, plus understanding, is needed for the beginning of recovery and redefinition. Difficult, but not entirely negative.

Disorientation occurs. Decisions are difficult and dependability is at great peril. There can even be the perception of a loss of IQ points. People can talk directly to us and we can react, but later, when called to carry out what we discussed or to remember something about the discussion, we can blank out completely and swear that the subject was never breached.

Tears sneak attack us when the bank teller asks for an endorsement from our dead spouse. We cry when someone bangs into our car in the parking lot and our spouse is not there to comfort us, yell at us, or handle the situation. We cry when the final doctor bills come in and we feel the insensitivity of the business world. We cry in front of our children, both a good and bad thing. It can frighten them but it can also give them permission to express their own emotions and it can show that we are human, capable of all emotions. We cry alone, in the privacy of our home. We cry with friends, and we can tell that the friends are getting tired of seeing the tears. Is it time to snap out of it? What if we start to cry and can't stop? What if we can't cry at all? What do friends and family think of us now and how do they think we are handling the situation? Do we care? Should we care? We are human, so we probably do. And they are probably at a loss as to what to say and how to help. And they might be frightened about the details of the death, and concerned that they might hurt us more by words and actions that might be seen as insensitive.

Individuals experiencing the death of a spouse will have varying degrees of trauma, all the way from mild to clinically severe. It can take a while to recover even from a mild trauma, and it takes work.

Identity. If we ever really know who we are, it is usually in the context of what others think of us and how successfully we interact with others, and especially with someone special. When we stay with someone for a long time and grow with each other, the two people can meld into an entity, a union. That entity consists of two individuals with hopes, fears, dreams, inter-linked in such a way that nothing is real unless the two people share the experience. This sharing can be argumentative as well as harmonious, but it is a sharing. The sharing is very human, and part of living life to the fullest. When the other person is gone, the link is gone, and with that, the framework or context is altered. Not only are we at a loss to bounce ideas off of someone, but also due to our weakened condition, we are forced to re-define all of our experiences, a distinct disadvantage.

In our case, after losing a large part of our identities, we set out to re-invent ourselves. We quickly learned that we were still who we used to be and decided to not re-invent, since we were not "invented" originally. The process of years of experiences and learning became the recipe of our personalities and with this event the process took a quantum leap. It is not so much re-inventing, as it is a process of the re-discovery of old things under a newer context, and discovery of new things. This could even lead to being a better person. We had to assimilate this leap as naturally as possible without over-intellectualizing.

So we must recover from a trauma and from the sadness associated with our spouse's fight. At some time it will be appropriate to start again, or restart our engines, whichever it takes.

OKAY, SO NOW WE REALLY BEGIN

PART ONE: GARY'S STORY

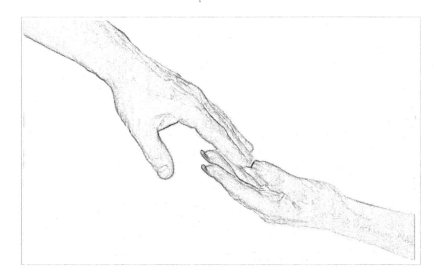

Chapter 1:
THE EARLY YEARS

The first thing you should know, to clear up confusion, is that my first wife was named *Kathie*, with an "*ie*" and my new wife is also named Kathy, but with a "y." This was always one of my favorite names, but this similarity was initially more of a negative than a positive for me. To help avoid the confusion, *Kathie's* name will be in italics and Kathy's will appear in regular font.

I met *Kathie* in 1967, at the University of Wisconsin in my third year of college and her first. She was turning eighteen and upon seeing her, I was turning cartwheels. She was the cutest thing that ever existed, bearing a resemblance to Katherine Ross. She had long, red hair with bangs, beautiful eyes of the darkest brown, exquisite bone structure in her face, beautiful, delicate fingers, about 5'2" and petite, with the cutest chapped lips ever. My first glimpse of her was in Spanish class. I bent over to pick up a dropped pencil and she was exiting the row. My eyes and her rear end met. That was fun, and it caught my attention. I was with her for twenty-two years after that moment.

Within months she took me home to St. Louis to meet the family. Five minutes into my visit, her nine-year-old brother asked me, "How much have you gotten off her?" I still rib him about that. Then I was served a two-layer cake, which slid off its moorings and onto her sister's foot. That took care of my nervousness.

Kathie was always a very quiet person, although she had no trouble communicating her feelings and thoughts, appropriate or not. She was not very good at sports and games frustrated her, even infuriated her. If she lost at a game, watch out! Her verbal wrath could be mighty. She was not a good loser. The only rages that I ever saw from her came from her frustration after losing a game. That may be partially why she fought so hard with the cancer, although she definitely did not see it as a game.

Kathie was very sensitive to the feelings of others and her own feelings were also quite acute, which often manifested as shyness. Because of this she was a private person with a small circle of friends. Her basic nature was very sweet with a finely tuned and readily available sense of humor. As *Kathie* grew more mature, she became very wise and her intelligence grew even more.

She was a very hard worker, perhaps too hard when it came to academic pursuits. She never settled for less than an A, and it took very hard work, but she always accomplished that. She attended graduate school during our early years. Her obsessiveness about schoolwork was a source of serious stress and conflict in our early marriage. The stress made her taciturn and negative toward me during those months, so much so that I was beginning to question whether or not I wanted to stay with her. I never talked about this to her because I sensed a metamorphosis happening with both of us, which soon led to our being even closer than before.

She earned her MBA with honors, and the behavioral anomalies were replaced by a glowing pregnancy, just at the right time.

Becoming a mother turned out to be the best therapy for *Kathie* because it gave her what she really wanted. I am doubly grateful for this because it enhanced the quality of both of our lives from that time forward.

Married life

I wrote, produced, directed, acted, applied for and received grants, did PR and swept floors for my non-profit touring theatre company. While building the foundation for the company, I made some wonderful friends.

Ellie

After seven years of staunch childlessness, we had a truly

inspired, "accidental" pregnancy, if you believe in accidents. I don't. Overnight, we were parents in every sense of the word. *Kathie* "popped the news" to me during the intermission of a Washington preview of the Jerry Lewis show "Hellzapoppin."

We were delirious and could not wait to tell family and friends, as well as anyone else who might listen. We speak of the "glow" that a pregnant woman has. *Kathie* and I both had that glow. We shared all of the doctor visits and the deliveries.

From the beginning, I knew what our first baby would look like and who she was. Now a grown woman, Ellie is a very sensitive, fun-loving, intense person. She loves to bring joy to others and has an extraordinary intuition about people.

I don't pretend to be objective about Ellie or our second "accidental" daughter, Robyn, and I'm glad that I had already learned to savor every good moment, because life with those children has been wonderful. These treasures would later help me through the hard times.

Both pregnancies went very well, with no morning sickness nor complications. *Kathie* breezed through so easily that she seemed to be invincible.

Kathie's **spiritual life**

Just prior to her illness, *Kathie* discovered NSA Buddhism. She felt a "rush" when she chanted. She felt that her original religious beliefs were not compromised. She considered the shrine that Buddhists use for chanting and meditation not an idol, but a means toward an ideal. I never embraced Buddhism, although I find the ideas surprisingly sensible. She found the chanting in combination with the philosophy perfect for her state of mind. This helped her marshal her strength for the fight of her life, soon to come.

Robyn

Kathie's second "accidental" pregnancy was greeted by total, unbridled enthusiasm. We told Ellie, then six, and she cried with joy. We taped the phone call telling my parents the good news. All five of us were on the phone. We don't listen to it much, but when we do, it is very strange to recall the joy, balanced with the early loss of *Kathie* and the moderately early loss of my father, who is also on the tape. But joy is joy, and we will take what we get, and milk it for every positive instant it brings.

Robyn was more of a mystery until she was born. She is a complete joy and a strong individual, with steadfast determination, ambition and strength. Later, an odd combination of Robyn's strength and her neediness helped me through the darkest times, along with Ellie's unconditional love and comfort. They both have a way of getting impatient with my less positive moments, reminding me always at the right time. They both know me well.

Our Good Fortune

Kathie nurtured me when I came down with pneumonia and when I sustained job-related injuries, teaching by example the quality of care that I would soon be called on to give to her.

Our family enjoyed a relatively idyllic life, punctuated with typical conflicts, frustrations and bickering. We were almost a cliché of urban/suburban bliss, *just waiting for the rug to be pulled out from under us.*

Chapter 2: ILLNESS

Discovery of the lump

What we could not know is that sometime between three and six years before diagnosis, *Kathie's* cancer had begun to slowly develop. A tumor such as this can be symptom and detection free for years.

Kathie had been breast-feeding Robyn for about six months in March of 1985, when I noticed an almond-size lump on the top of her left breast, a few inches down from the clavicle.

At the doctor's office two days later, the doctor palpated the lump and with confidence told us it was probably a milk cyst, a common occurrence for a lactating woman. He made an appointment for an aspiration to relieve the pressure and vent the milk, which should have eliminated the cyst.

Everyone was surprised and more than a little alarmed that the aspiration produced no results. That meant that it was a tumor, but breast feeding women "never" have cancer, so the next step was suggested almost in a light hearted manner. Conservative medicine dictated a biopsy.

We went into the biopsy really expecting nothing exciting. Women who have breast-fed are statistically less prone to breast cancer, and here was a woman *currently* breast-feeding. They anesthetized *Kathie* and I waited outside. As I was waiting alone with my thoughts, my fears surfaced and inwardly I started to panic a little bit. The procedure was taking longer than I was led to expect, so my mind started to conjure up some scary stuff.

Finally the doctor came out with a stunned look on his

face. It was cancer. I felt a tremendous heat and an unheard explosion. Regaining my composure some, I began to formulate how I was going to tell *Kathie*. I had never dealt with anything like this and felt totally unprepared. The doctor must have seen this on my face. He had already told her and she was dealing with it, better than I.

In the recovery room, she was a little groggy, quiet, and withdrawn. She said she knew, and that it could be handled, already showing her strength and determination, teaching me the first of many lessons. She was calm, accepting, and ready to deal with it. This was an abrupt change of gears from the elation of having a new baby to the prospect of having a potentially long, debilitating and possibly fatal illness. *Kathie* chose to focus on the positive things around her, such as her new baby, and she set out to win. I changed gears outwardly to a more positive mode. I was still screaming inside.

Ultimately, her spirituality and my support helped garner her resources and focus on the healing.

We sought a second opinion and began contemplation. A modified radical mastectomy was prescribed, for which *Kathie* would have to stop breast-feeding "cold turkey." We had been supplementing Robyn with a little formula every day, so this was a little easier than it might have been. They remained very close throughout their short four and one-half years together.

Kathie was given some medication to dry up the breast milk, because the operation could not be done while the vessels were engorged with blood. She was outwardly reasonably okay about losing the breast and having reduction on the other. "I wanted reduction surgery anyway," she said. Of course, it was hard for her even though she was not very verbal about it.

She was very clear about the loss of her breast. It was necessary in order to live. *Kathie* was my wife, the mother of my children, and the best part of my own identity so, of course, I never found her any less desirable without the breast. She knew me well, so she understood that. I was just glad to have her with me.

While on the phone, telling our parents about the cancer, my mind flashed to the taped phone conversation about eighteen months earlier, announcing *Kathie's* pregnancy to the family. Same type of setting this time, but the other side of life's surprises.

Taking charge

The operation took about four hours, without complications. Her side lymph nodes were clear and the lump appeared to be contained. The tumor turned out to be estrogen negative and ductile, occurring within the milk ducts, neither factor being the best sign for a pre-menopausal woman. But we were told not to be overly worried because of the clean margins.

Actually, *Kathie* had many bad signs for re-growth. The nodes on her side were negative, but there are other nodes, especially just above the site of the tumor, about two inches down from the clavicle on the left side. These nodes were not routinely checked in 1985. With the tumor so close to those nodes, one would think that they should have been checked, but they were not. I don't know if it would have made a difference at the time, but that did turn out to be the site of the return.

Still, we were told that the odds, based on medical knowledge in 1985, were considered to be good. With the knowledge that I have now, I would have tried hard to find a way to continue the chemotherapy, even if with a different blend of agents.

Kathie decided that she would have reconstructive surgery, rather than wear a prosthesis. A second operation would be required for a tissue expander and a third for the implant and an adjustment to the other breast for symmetry. She had one breast reconstructed, with a new nipple, and had a reduction in the other one. The results were good, although not entirely like the real thing. The breast was hard and sensation only partially returned to that area, due to the nerves that were severed during the mastectomy. She handled it stoically.

At this point, the prudent and conservative course of action was adjuvant chemotherapy. A combination of 5fluorouracil, methotrexate and cytoxan was used. She was offered an ice cap, which sometimes retards the loss of hair, but she found it very uncomfortable, and elected to drop it.

The first treatment was sneaky. Chemo agents were administered about 11:00 A.M. She felt fine and ate a large dinner. Around 11:00 P.M. she began to vomit, which continued all night. The next day she was listless, but the vomiting passed after she took a dosage of compazine to relieve the nausea. Spending the day in bed, half awake, she had a lot of time to think. I don't know how, but she managed to channel her resources, and even though she was exceptionally tired, she was well the next day.

She lost her hair, and was very upbeat about a condition that devastates many people. She reasoned that anything that made her better was worth a temporary loss of hair, showing her strength and ability to put things into perspective. She bought a beautiful wig, which looked quite natural.

Her body did not like the chemotherapy. Her strength was completely zapped and the need for rest was insatiable for several miserable days. There were dark circles under her eyes. The fatigue offered opportunities for the fear of the disease and fear of the unknown to creep into her mind. Chemo is a rude slap in the face, a wake-up call, which says, "Hey, you have cancer. Deal with it!"

The second dose, a few weeks later, produced a similar, but noticeably stronger reaction.

The third dose produced a dangerous reaction and at 1:00 A.M. we sped to an emergency room, with *Kathie* seemingly near death from irregular heartbeat, uncontrolled vomiting and general panic. *Kathie* recovered enough that night to be allowed to go home, and returned to normal within a week. Due to the escalating danger of the reactions, we were only able to do only three of the six chemotherapy treatments. The literature at the time said that only five percent of these tumors returned, and the expected recurrence was equal with or without the chemo. Conservative medicine dictated the course, "just in case."

Her blood family was as supportive as possible, but they were separated by thousands of miles and health and dependency concerns at home.

We spent a year dealing with the illness and its diagnosis, the mastectomy, the chemotherapy, and the reconstruction. *Kathie's* energy was shot, but she slowly began to recover and started to lead a normal life. Yes, it was like life on a banana peel. Every illness or ache was interpreted as a possible cancer.

Despite all of this, she took up horseback riding and we took frequent vacations. Since could not be sure what the outcome of her cancer would be, we had fun and did interesting things, and she purchased some things that might have been rejected under different circumstances. We were both fatalistic and optimistic, but we were certain that it would be stupid turn down opportunities.

Among the fun things was *Kathie's* idea to attend Club Med in Guadalupe. It was beautiful and memorable. One thing really surprised me. *Kathie* took us to a Club Med nude beach. We had never done such a thing, and most people probably wouldn't. If she had warned me beforehand, I probably would have chickened out. But here we were at a nude beach, and *Kathie* had just had reconstructive surgery. She took it in stride. If she could handle it, I surely should be able to handle it. So I mellowed into it as we parked ourselves under a tree, occasionally wading into the warm, green waters. No jellyfish, fortunately!

We were two of an international crowd of probably 1000 naked people, mostly families, on a mile and a half of beach, so things quickly settled down to sameness, surprisingly non-sexual. I did not find it very sexy, except privately with *Kathie*, as if we had a little secret. So it was fun.

The next day, we called home to check on things and heard that my father had suffered a seizure. Upon our return to the states two days later, I rushed to Florida where my father was undergoing an exploratory procedure for a brain tumor. It turned out to be inoperable. He broke the news to me, but I already had been told by the doctors. I think they should have coordinated that with him, so he would not have felt the burden of telling me.

"I'm gonna let you down this time," he said. "The doctors give me six months. I say four." He was right. He gradually lost the use of his body and mind and died in four months.

California/Second Lump

In 1986 *Kathie* convinced me to consider a move to southern California.

After one week in California, my father died of the brain tumor. I could not cry, even though it would have been a good thing. The need was there, yet a strange father/son combination of anger, conditioning, frustration, and incompleteness made the event seem emotionally remote. Perhaps I had not grown emotionally mature enough to allow myself to deal with it at that time. I did have a full emotional plate dealing with all of the issues surrounding *Kathie's* illness.

Kathie's health seemed to hold up fairly well during the second year after the operations and chemo.

We moved to Los Angeles in August of 1987, about six months after *Kathie* began to show some troubling symptoms.

Her left shoulder was achy. The mastectomy was on that side. She thought, or hoped, that the pain was related to a tugging incident with Robyn, then three years old. It was a minor candy struggle and had absolutely nothing to do with the pain.

It's interesting, what you remember. Ten years later, while talking to Robyn, she revealed that she had always thought the shoulder pain and subsequent illness and death was due to that tugging incident. Imagine going through life thinking that!

Kathie was in denial. Who wouldn't be? The chemo almost killed her the first time, so the prospect of a second round had to be unfathomable.

The shoulder got progressively more painful. We went to our first Los Angeles oncologist who neglected to take routine frozen blood samples, therefore missing detection of the enzyme that clearly signifies a return of breast cancer. He also dismissed the ache and a new lump that I had discovered, as an adhesion related to the mastectomy. This was a truly stupid and life-threatening misdiagnosis. I knew he was wrong and tried very hard to talk *Kathie* into doing something proactive about the pain, more than just taking aspirin. David, her physician brother, also worked hard to try to convince her. She changed oncologists and ended up with a truly gifted group, but it was too late. The year of denial and misdiagnosis had taken its toll.

After *Kathie* died, we were in no emotional condition to sue the first oncologist, even though the thought occurred. After a period of time, I approached my attorney for his advice. He informed me that there was a statute of limitations but there was no hurry to decide on a course of action. The money could have been useful for the children, but I am not the litigating type, and this type of suit can be hard to prove, so I waited until I was stronger. It turned out that my attorney's advice was in error, and the statute ran out significantly earlier than he thought. Now my attorney was open to a malpractice suit. Many people said that I should have sued him, but I wanted to concentrate on the children with a positive utilization of my limited energies.

I finally talked *Kathie* into seeing a neurologist. Nerve conductivity tests were performed to see the extent of the nerve involvement and, in a sneaky way, to suggest whether or not it may be a true tumor. His test showed a high level of nerve involvement. This doctor was the first responsible physician other than her brother to see the site of the lump. His face dropped and went ashen, unprepared for such horrible results from a young woman. His face betrayed what he could not ethically say to us. The oncologist should have acted on this a long time ago.

After the appointment, we discussed the doctor's reaction. After deciding that he was probably a bad poker player, with a little ironic chuckle, *Kathie* took it as a concrete warning, pulled herself out of denial, and took action. And she told me that if we were ever to play poker, this doctor should be invited.

The treatment

The new oncologists took the frozen blood specimen and found the enzyme that indicates metastasized breast cancer. That is, breast cancer that has recurred either in the breast area, or any other area of the body. The tumor was probed for cells that would more conclusively tell whether or not cancer was present. The tumor was so hard and compact that it was difficult to retrieve the cells utilizing a minimally invasive procedure. But they succeeded. They performed further tests, which identified many small sites in the lungs and referred *Kathie* to radiation for the lump, now about walnut size. She was also referred to a MRI lab to more specifically pinpoint the lesions in the lungs, and to see if there were any other surprises.

Radiation began with a small temporary tattoo, marking the target for the radiologist. The radiologist was surprisingly verbal in her criticism of *Kathie's* first Los Angeles oncologist.

Inevitable burning from the radiation caused scarring on her lungs. The large tumor was the only spot specifically radiated, but there is always residual burning, scarring, and discomfort, to a greater or lesser degree, depending on the case. She had eight treatments.

Our optimism, already tempered with doses of reality, turned pessimistic and a quiet panic set in. Much was left unsaid by *Kathie,* who did not want to talk about her illness. One day, about a year before her death, we were talking about a cottage in the mountains that we had considered purchasing in a few years. *Kathie* said that she would probably never see it. I tried to reassure her, but I am sure that I could not completely hide my pessimism. At that time, she also had difficulty retrieving that old optimism.

The MRI is a non-invasive, radiation-free test that images soft tissues by using a magnetic field. The images are very detailed and give cross sections like a CT scan.

As non-invasive as the test is, if you have claustrophobia, which *Kathie* had, it can be frightening. This MRI was like a very small tunnel or tube, just big enough to fit a person. A conveyer belt slowly carried her through, inch by inch. After a few seconds of imaging, she came out for a little breather. The walls were right in her face and she was totally submerged in its workings even though both ends are wide open. The noise of the MRI is also a startling, banging sound. *Kathie* felt like she was in a coffin and got very panicky. I held her hand as much as was allowed, and that helped. The whole process took about forty-five minutes. Some of the newer MRI's are doughnut-shaped, eliminating the claustrophobia.

The test results are read and passed along to the doctor, but the results are immediate. No processing is required. The technicians reacted with alarm, especially given her age. Not knowing that we knew about *Kathie's* lung involvement, they tried to use their poker faces, but shock, alarm, and sadness was written all over their faces.

There were lesions everywhere. Small, but pervasive. That would make chemotherapy very tricky. *Kathie* was breathing hard and coughing, due to Pneumonitis, which we thought was brought about by the radiation therapy. In hindsight, Pneumonitis was only part of the culprit. The lung lesions that had been slow growing at first, really did most of the damage when they unexpectedly started growing rapidly.

The MRI confirmed the extent of the involvement and hinted that there were other organs showing abnormalities. Chemotherapy, radiation, heavy Buddhist chanting, and as much physical healing as I could conjure, were the chosen tools. I would have studied and recommended the addition of holistic therapies if we had more time. The doctors were cognizant of her reaction to the chemo the first time, so they prescribed a light course, once a week, with close monitoring.

She expected to lose her hair again, so we ordered a beautiful wig at a store near our home, which she did not live to wear.

Kathie suffered through many months of difficulty catching her breath, with a persistent cough. It was exhausting for her and very troubling to see. She was prescribed several forms of codeine for cough control, but the medicine was ineffective. Her color remained good, however, which means that *just* enough oxygen was getting through. Her activities were greatly curtailed.

The first and last dose

The first dose of chemo seemed to go fairly well at first. She did not get overly nauseous and it looked like she would tolerate it well. But the chemo caused the many small lung lesions to swell, choking off her oxygen supply, causing a crisis. This cure unexpectedly led to her death. No one thought that her life would be in such serious danger so early. We expected that she would be able to control the disease for the eight to ten years, barring any new discovery that would extend it further.

Several days after that first dose, she was chanting in our living room with three of her NSA friends, louder and more forcefully than I had ever heard. At the end, the chanters went home. After they were gone, *Kathie* was unable to catch her breath. The optimism of the chanting had turned into a barely controlled panic. We arrived at the oncologist's office in about twenty minutes. They took her immediately, much faster than if we had chosen an emergency room and an ambulance. They set her up with oxygen, which at that point helped only a little. The discomfort was one thing, but the oxygen deprivation induced claustrophobia and she became very frightened.

The waiting room was packed with patients waiting for administration of chemotherapy. They saw what was happening to this young lady, and needless to say, everyone's eyes were wide.

The hospital was in the next building. The doctor saw to it that her emergency admittance to the hospital next door went smoothly and rapidly. One of the doctor's assistants quickly wheeled *Kathie* to the hospital, and immediately into the Cardiac Care Unit, which is like an intensive care unit. She was given both an oxygen tube and a mask. A nurse often came in to stick her finger for blood gas readings. Really uncomfortable. Her appetite was gone and her limbs became impossibly heavy. She could not even raise her arms.

I stayed at the hospital all day, returning home only to be with the children at night and put them to bed.

Her family came in from New Jersey and St. Louis, recognizing that this was no ordinary setback.

We both had a long list of fears and concerns, mostly unspoken. *Kathie* knew what she was going through as she struggled to breathe. She feared death and the unknown.

After the first day, the oncologist assigned a pulmonary specialist and an infectious disease specialist, to be sure all the bases were covered, but the diagnosis was obvious. The chemo had taken its toll in a striking way. The dramatic change was not only her reaction to the chemo, through swelling of the lung tissues, but also the sudden change in the cancer, going from a very slow-growing condition to an explosive growth situation.

At the end of the first day, the oncologist pulled me aside and told me that we should hope that she had a form of pneumonia, for which they were giving her "guerillamicin," a slang for a powerful, full spectrum antibiotic. If it was not pneumonia, she would probably never return home. That was another bolt of lightning. I knew how desperate she had become in those last many hours, but I was not at all prepared to hear such a dire warning.

The nursing staff was heroic. I really felt for them because they were doing their jobs efficiently and professionally, in spite of the obvious emotion that they were feeling.

Kathie and I passed the time trying hard to be positive and trying to concentrate our focus on healing. I read to her because it was nearly impossible for her to speak, and many times I just sat there with her.

The family behaved well, with love and caring, showing strength and unity. Prior to this, they had been unaware that her cancer had returned, so for them it was an even bigger shock. *Kathie* had chosen to hold off telling her family and friends until

she began to lose her hair due to the chemo, which had not yet occurred. She was concerned that people would categorize her as a
cancer patient or a dying person or a curiosity, and wanted to delay that as long as possible. She also wanted to limit any negativity that might hinder the healing process, by hindering uninterrupt-
ed concentration. She knew that her mind was the biggest healer,
so she needed to be as positive as possible. This emergency inter-
vened and changed everything.

Inevitably, the family pointed a few fingers at me, asking,
"Why didn't you tell us?" But they soon became satisfied that it
was *Kathie's* wish, not mine, that she undertake this journey alone.
They still wished that they could have known earlier. I would
have welcomed support earlier. I needed help. The burden of the
illness and its implications was unrelenting on both of us.

Kathie was truly happy to see them and benefited immensely by their presence. At first, with events happening so suddenly and with such surprise, I was really not sure whether or not to
call them. She had been so forceful and clear in her admonition to
keep the secret. Her condition was desperate. I didn't want her
to hate me, especially at this moment, but it was the best thing.
Even if she hated me for it, it would still be better for her to have
her family there.

The family support set the scene for a stronger bond than
ever between them, my family, and ultimately my new Kathy.

On the fourth day, in desperate shape, she still expressed
an amazing determination to win. Robyn and Ellie visited and
saw her somewhat stronger and more alert than during previous
days. Was this a sign that things were turning around? There
was the slightest glimmer of hope, contrary to all signs and logic,
that the guerillamicin might have started to take effect and that
the condition was a treatable pneumonia after all. *Kathie* expressed love and interest in the children's activities. The visit was
short and the children came away with the definite feeling that
their mom was in real trouble, but that it was not hopeless. The
tubes could have been frightening to the children, so we introduced
the "outer space" gadgets carefully. Her color was fairly good, so
she did not look as bad as she actually was.

A lung biopsy would have told us whether or not it was
pneumonia, but that would have required an invasive procedure

and in her delicate condition, she would have had to be hooked up to a respirator. *Kathie* clearly prohibited anything that would put her in this position. She felt that if things were that bad, it would just prolong the agony and make things harder for everyone.

It was not pneumonia. She had been in the hospital five sleepless and frightening nights and days when she had endured all she could take. Gathering what breath she could muster, she talked to me about her fear during her fourth sleepless night. It was very hard for her to be alone, even for a second. I decided to stay all night from then on, which turned out to be only one night. As she began to come to grips with the dying process, her philosophy about life did not waver, regardless of the fear. Dying was part of life, regardless of when it might happen. Her personal picture of an afterlife was still in the formulation stages, but she definitely believed that there was something afterward, whether it was reincarnation or some other form.

I knew nothing about funeral arrangements, but I was forced to think about what to do and how to find information. The only thing I knew of *Kathie's* wishes is that she wanted to be cremated. When I tried to find out if she had any other requests or needs, she wanted nothing of it and said, "Deal with it." I did.

But I thought, "Me in charge?"

She had been unable to lift her arms for about twenty-four hours, but gathered strength from somewhere. Something told her that it was the end. I don't know exactly how she knew, but she did. Looking amazingly beautiful, *Kathie* called us in, one-by-one. With a halting and painful but caring breath, she told each of us that she loved us and said good-bye.

And when *Kathie* and I were alone, true to her Buddhist philosophy, she said her last words, " It's natural. It's part of life. I'll always be with you, and I love you."

And that is true.

Everyone cried, including the nursing staff. Suffice it to say, there wasn't a dry eye for the next eighteen hours until her death and afterward. But we did have "closure." Many people do not have a final moment with their spouse, especially if there is a sudden death. Also, old communication problems can get in the way and sabotage such a moment. This closure helped me to cope with the realities in a setting that seemed more dream-like than real. This is the kind of dream I desperately needed to wake up from, but never did.

Kathie strongly requested an additional drip of morphine. She had a profound need for rest and peace. She was aware that she was dying and that the morphine might suppress her respiration further, perhaps causing death a little sooner, but she had no choice. She was hours away from death in any case, and she was desperate for relief.

The drip was started and she immediately felt better. Before her last words she told me that she was feeling peaceful, relieved, and less frightened. During this episode, physical touch had been uncomfortable to her, but now she asked me to hold her hand. She drifted off and I let go only to eat a little snack and to go to the bathroom. Her brother or sister held her hand during my brief absences.

For the next eighteen hours, after she fell into the coma, I talked with the family members, who gathered around her, and I talked to *Kathie*. I don't know if she heard me. She was determined to die with dignity, just as she had fought the illness. This is why I say that she won the battle with cancer. This was a real lesson for me. I told her she was doing great and that we were with her.

She was almost completely "out of it" during this time. The nurses came in to try to catheterize her, but even in her comatose state, catheterization was uncomfortable for her and she resisted, making faces and noises. Her kidneys had shut down by then, so it was unnecessary to push it. She had a similar reaction as the nurses cleared mucus a few times. Even through the process of dying, her body was clinging to life. She even started her period during that time. And it was a normal one at exactly the right time. I was amazed.

The nurses stayed close by, but gave the family space. *Kathie's* heartbeat began to slow. One of the nurses gently told me that the end was here. I held *Kathie's* hand and watched the heart monitor (the sound had been turned off) as it slowed down. My feelings about the near-death or approaching death experiences are mixed, but you never know, so I looked to the ceiling and spoke to her, said goodbye and waved, just in case she was up there, hovering. I told her that I loved her and that she would always be there in my heart. Then the monitor stopped and I knew.

Even after all the anticipation and preparation, my body went limp and I fell to my knees, crying loudly. My brother in law, Ron, caught me and held me. I looked at *Kathie* and then the monitor. Then it started again. Was this the start of a recovery? Even then I had a glimmer of hope that things could improve. Confusion and anger, combined with desperate sadness. What was this? It turned out to be a momentary extra beat or two, followed by quiet.

I looked up to the ceiling and tried to smile and wave. I might have felt stupid for a second, but it was something that we had talked about, so if she was up there, I didn't want to miss the opportunity. If she was not up there, I really didn't have a problem looking stupid. I was getting good at it.

Chapter 3: DYING

Sounds terribly harsh, doesn't it? Not surprisingly, I had quite a bit of trouble coming to grips with that. Saying it out loud hurt terribly but helped me to come to reality, a concept that was about to be in short supply.

There is no easy way to talk about the process of dying. Everyone has to go through it and at some point everyone becomes a survivor of someone close. But it never gets easy, especially with those you love.

The moment of death came. I would like to say that it came and went, but when it came, it stayed with me for a long time. The preparations for grief probably started subconsciously the instant that she was first diagnosed, four years earlier, became more immediate after the re-diagnosis, and intensified after the emergency admission to the hospital.

But no degree of anticipation would prepare me for the moment when it came. It was not sudden. It was not a shock, even though the end was a surprise, earlier and more abrupt than we had anticipated. It progressed in an almost linear way. And yet, the effect was total shock.

I didn't want to let her go. I wanted my life to continue with her. Life without her seemed ludicrous. But my wonderful daughters, gave me a reason, motivation and the courage and strength to go on. Despite my fatalistic state, my children enabled me to begin to see the possibilities for the future.

Prior to her death, thinking that I was more tenacious than I really was, I had thought that my primary mourning would be short, due to my preparation throughout the stages of her illness. But my mourning was more protracted than I had "planned" for, and no enlightenment, conscious or otherwise, conditioned me for the reality of her passing. The genuine mourning had not begun earlier and I had received no effective preparation. It was a whole new ball game. It felt like the bottom of the ninth with the bases loaded and the odds against me. It would take a grand slam to get me out of this state of mind.

The tearful call to the mortuary put the wheels in motion.

I had been mindful that there was not much time left for us during those last days, so I had cherished holding her hand and looking at her face as much as possible. She was a bit gaunt, but the final course of the disease hit so suddenly that her appearance never looked moribund. Now she was gone, and I looked at her for the last time, and kissed her. Her face was beginning to feel cool, which only added to the strangeness and the sadness. I thanked the nurses, and made it out to my car, alone.

Kathie was gone. We had been so much a part of each other that it felt like my identity was gone, and it continued feeling that way for a long time.

The time tunnel

When *Kathie* was sick, I wanted the time to go fast, so that we would have an assurance that the cancer was finished. Now that she was gone, I wished that the time had gone more slowly so that I could feel like I had her for a longer time.

My recovery time seemed to go slowly, but I certainly didn't want that. Looking back now after more than ten years, it feels like it went more quickly than I perceived at the time, but I'm glad to be on this side of it. Now, as I grow older, I am happy to let time to go as slowly as possible, in a perfect world, that is.

Driving Home

I drove home with tears in my eyes, which was challenging and very dangerous. Don't try this. Get help. People will do the driving for you. Later, in my support group, many others recounted how they had to drive home alone after the death, through tears. In one of many moments of black comedy, the support group members determined that death can be hazardous to your health. It might seem stupid to drive alone, but neither logic nor options were anywhere near me at the time.

Between the tears, aware of the danger, I drove very carefully. It was particularly important for me to arrive home alive for the children. And it was time to tell the children.

Crying

My father was a strict disciplinarian with some old ideas. When you are a boy, you do not cry. "Crying is for sissies." My story is similar to many children of my age. One day I fried my hand in bacon grease and received first, second, and third degree burns. I was ten, so I cried. My father said, "Stop crying or I'll give you something to cry about." The mind boggles. A typical macho, 1950's type philosophy. My subconscious must have told me, "If this is not good enough to cry about, then I guess nothing is." That was my last real cry for thirty-three years. Sadly, when my father died, I still could not cry.

My father never let me show emotions, even though in later years, he became very emotional, an irony that was not lost on me. Yes, he contributed in large measure to my difficulty, inadvertently teaching me to mistrust my inner truth and my emotions, and that conditioning made it hard to cry when he died. Also, other emotional scars from childhood, some very subtle, had heightened my defenses. It took many years to realize that I am responsible for my own emotional life, and blame is unproductive.

This essential component of my emotional life returned with *Kathie's* death, bringing me closer to my definition of human, the hard way. A believer in the healing power of tears, I was acutely aware of the loss of the ability to cry and was ready for its return. That is the crux of the issue: permission to be completely honest with my own feelings, and the knowledge that I am better for having them. Surprisingly, I was always able to fully enjoy the emotion and expression of love.

When the tears started, they came forcefully. No, this onslaught did not scare me. I had been ready for a long time. I can't say that it felt good to cry, but the tears were beneficial, and I know that if I had not cried at this time, I would probably have had the equivalent of a complete breakdown.

The good news is that I was fully expressing the emotion,

and as sad as the circumstances were, it felt healthy, like survival.

Ironically, the day I cried, the day *Kathie* died, I became liberated from emotional insecurity (mostly), now able to leap tall life experiences with a single bound. I now cry appropriately (my definition of appropriately) and always will from now on.

The bad news is that *Kathie* saw me cry on her last day of life. She had never seen me cry, so that was an indescribable moment for her. She was facing the end of her life and she was fearful of the unknown, so my tears caused her great difficulty.

"I'm sorry," she said, struggling to get any words out at all. This is probably a natural thing to feel, but I felt so much sadder for her because of her need to apologize.

That triggered the crying.

Very awkwardly, I said, "You really shouldn't apologize. If anything, I'm the one who should apologize..." I didn't really finish the sentence but burst into tears for the first time since I was ten. Her tone went from apologetic to angry.

"Stop crying. You shouldn't cry."

She felt that my tears were detrimental, working against her energy to fight the disease. Recalling a familiar aphorism from my childhood, that was the least appropriate thing anyone could say to me at that time. *Kathie* and I had spoken occasionally about my inability to cry and she had shown that she clearly approved of tears, in theory anyway. I did not express the anger that I felt upon hearing those words, and continued the crying, which, fortunately for me, could not be helped. I also understood her point of view. But I had no choice. And that was good. I was evolving into a better human being, the hard way. If my wife's death wasn't a reason to cry, then what was? And it was a universe worse than the bacon grease from my childhood.

When she apologized for her condition I was thunderstruck. What do you say? I didn't want her to feel even worse. Not only was she faultless, but she had done everything in her power to make things better. Her long denial upon the first signs of the recurrence was the reaction of a frightened human being.

I must admit, I did fault her for the denial, but I also understood what she was facing. I do feel that the crying may have in some small way supported her acceptance of the end.

During this "new" experience of crying, I accidentally saw

myself in a mirror in the hospital room and it looked just as strange as I thought it would.

Months later, I found my emotional limits.

Some people are worried that if they start to cry they will never stop. It can feel that way. But you stop, eventually, if only to sleep. People take as much time to process each phase of their grief as they need. There is no formula, contrary to some popular folklore. (see Appendix B: Timetable for Grief)

My children had also never seen me cry. Crying in this context is normal and expected, but strange for children to witness. It makes them feel insecure. It connotes the loss, even temporary, of the parent's power, even considering the perceived downside of strict parenting. Even though my children knew that it was proper and expected, my tears were a little alienating and frightening, and for a while it happened often. However, we could always see the absurdity, so we often had a caustic comment at the ready.

It is also good for the children to see the adults cry. It shows that the parent is human and it gives the child permission to grieve and evolve his or her recovery from loss, at his or her own speed. My children and I always communicated well, so after some months, my children were confident that they could suggest that it was time to stop. I took that as a signal and a friendly slap in the face. I was going to have to put a genuine effort into my recovery from grief.

Laughing

Laughing? *Kathie* had just died. I was enduring the saddest, most desperate time of my life. I was crying much of the time. Laughing? Laughter is a healer. When I regained my sense of humor, I took an important step toward reclaiming control, and resuscitating normalcy. This is a new definition of normalcy, to be sure, but as valid as the normalcy perceived prior to the illness and death.

What's so funny, anyway? Strange things. A spontaneous moment might strike me the right way. I might go to a purely "escapist" movie, or maybe a comedy club to get "out of my head," as people used to call it.

Here is an example of laughter as an island within a mass

of tears. It seems that each event leading up to *Kathie's* death and many events surrounding it and after it were all the "hardest thing I've ever done." The most formidable of those "hardest things" was telling my children that their mother had died.

We were upstairs in a loft area, away from the gathering family downstairs. Robyn, age five, was on my left and Ellie, age twelve, was on my right, with our pet Boxer, Cookie, a little more to the right. We had been crying hard for about fifteen minutes. Then Cookie let out a very strange sound. It sounded like a combination of a yawn/howl/"aw stop it" mix. The only time in her life she ever did that particular sound. The odd timing made it very funny. We each went from crying hard to laughing hard for about thirty seconds. We had a brief respite. A chance to catch our emotional breath. Then we went back to crying hard. This was a small moment, but I'm convinced that it had strong healing power. It was a ridiculous sound, a reaction at our expressions of distress. It also worked for her, because we embraced her and included her in the very sad, private moment.

It was a while before I wanted to see a comedy show or listen to jokes, but once it happened, within a few weeks, it felt good, if strange at first. I needed to wallow in the sadness full-time for a while, until I was ready to accept healing. During most of my life, I have possessed humor at the ready, sometimes appropriately, sometimes not. So it was relatively easy to rediscover wit. Some people are not as fortunate, and experience a combination of grief and depression, which can preclude the ability to laugh or enjoy in the face of the great loss recently suffered.

Telling the children: the hardest thing I have ever done
Handling the children during the illness, and now especially after *Kathie's* death, was the most important responsibility, and the hardest thing that I have ever done. With one unfortunate turn of a phrase, I could traumatize them. I was determined to help them through this and try to make it easier. The children would need to be cherished more than ever, for their sake and also for mine. I was reminded that soon enough they would also leave the nest. Their tenure with me would be temporary due to the natural growing up process. I was thinking ahead and already missing them. Life is full of the temporary and full of interruptions. I

wanted their temporary time with me to be as rich as possible. Years later, at Ellie's high school graduation, it all came into focus. I felt this transition and cried through the *entire* ceremony. No, I didn't make a scene, but I really had a hard time of it. On the other hand, I reminded myself that if I raised them the right way, they would become their own person and voluntarily leave the nest.

How do you tell a child that her mother is seriously ill? How do you tell a child that her mother might die, or probably would die? How do you tell a child that her mother has died? I'm a believer in logic, instinct, love, sensitivity, careful study of exactly who the children are, and ultimately, "punting." All of those qualities went into my presentations, but I never really knew if I was doing good or harm until afterwards. Later, I found that my instincts were right in one area. I was careful to characterize the death as sad and unwelcome but natural. I didn't want to make heaven seem so beautiful that a young child might get any ideas of joining her mom. It does happen. Also, I did not tell the children that their mom was asleep. Some children develop a fear of sleeping if they hear that. It seems to soften the impact of death, but it can make the child fearful of not waking up. Also, it gives some children false hope that their parent might wake up, and nightmares of the parent awakening inside the coffin.

The children knew that *Kathie's* death was probably imminent, so it was not a complete shock, but no less sad for knowing that it was coming. We held out hope that healing would occur until the very last second. The death represents a loss and also the end of a battle, with the immediate perception of losing the battle as well as a strange peacefulness recognizing that her suffering has ended.

My language with the children would be as it had always been, careful but direct, including tone of voice, eye contact, body language, and setting in this equation. Before I could speak, the message was communicated from my body language, from the way the events were transpiring, and from activity surrounding the gathering of people downstairs, but I still had to tell them. So I looked into their faces as they waited for the news that they dreaded, ending the uncertainty. *Kathie's* decision to put off telling the children about the recurrence of cancer made this harder, given the sudden explosion of the illness. But the children saw what she had been going through during those last days and months, and must have known more than they were consciously able to accept.

"Mom passed away this morning."

A brief silence was punctuated by each of us crying hard and embracing. After a while, the questions came. "When? Were you there? Was she in pain? Who else was there? Are we going to St. Louis to be with mom's side of the family?" Neither *Kathie*, myself, or the children ever asked, "Why me?" But I did hear, "Why her?" This question came from everyone, especially from me. I knew that there was no answer for such a question, but human nature caused me to ask anyway.

Our closeness helped immensely. We talked about *Kathie's* life, about our intangible feelings of receiving her life energy at the end, about looking up and waving, and how beautiful she looked even at the end. We cried hard and long with each other. Then we went about our tasks of helping each other pack to go to St. Louis. We apparently packed our bags well, leaving nothing out, but I don't remember doing it.

My journey begins

At this moment I perceived the first inkling that my life had been changed profoundly. Who was I? It suddenly dawned on me. I was a widower. A new label. I would have to struggle to find myself again. Before this, I really knew myself, and now I was foundering.

I felt profound, all-encompassing sadness. *Kathie's* fight was over, but I felt tremendous sorrow that she had to endure such pain, especially at such a young age. And I was sad that she would never see the development of her children. I felt equally sad for my children, so young, who no longer had a mother, a loss especially dear since *Kathie* was such a loving and active mom.

The arrangements

Kathie chose not to discuss dying and her death came suddenly, leaving me somewhat unprepared. I only knew that she wanted to be cremated. That much was clear because we had talked about it many times, and it was specified in her will. We both strongly believed in God, and we are definitely spiritual people, but we were not very religiously observant, our beliefs being more practical, secular and personal. When the family asked to have her wishes overridden, I refused, but feeling for their loss and their emotional state, I compromised on all other conditions, since *Kathie* had not specifically declared them.

Her family would have wanted her to have a traditional burial, contrary to her own beliefs.

The cemetery, where many of the spouses from my support group are buried, is in Burbank, next to the celebrity populated Forest Lawn. There were a few options, but the cost, timing and procedures were all packaged. Fewer options at a time like that present an upside and a downside. It is a business, after all, but one requiring sensitivity, as well as intuitive and logical thinking on the part of the salesperson.

I was not handled well. I knew to anticipate financial problems brought about by hospitalization and loss of income. Most survivors have that concern. In my emotional state I never thought to ask the mortuary representative if there were any payment plans. The package was presented as a dollar amount, due immediately, with no hint to the contrary. I should have questioned this, and I would have if I were not deluged by emotions, which clouded my thinking. I was in a fog, like so many others in the same circumstance. It would have been wise and kind of the salesperson to suggest that payment plans were available.

My stepfather and *Kathie's* father joined me and were very helpful making the funeral arrangements.

Every family member was very sensitive and giving. Not every family reacts this way. Some of my young widow and widower friends and acquaintances have told me horror stories about family rifts that surfaced at this moment, as well as other moments during the emotionally charged days preceding and following the death. My mother and my stepfather, who is really a dad to me, were trying to shield me, as parents do, and continue to actively support and counsel. *Kathie's* family members, who I love, are true, honest and caring. I felt badly for their loss as well and I felt badly that I could not come to their aid. They came to my aid, but I was consumed by my emotions, so even though I was aware of their pain, I was not as healing for them as I would have liked.

I have been described as a "caretaker" type. So it is not unusual that I would feel some responsibility for the family's recovery. And that is quite proper, but one cannot always assume the caretaker role. At this particular time, I needed to be "caretaken" myself, if that is a word I may coin. I had never been very good at accepting help. Accepting help and giving in to this need was a major step for me, and a sneaky sign of human growth.

The oak and brass casket, which her father chose, was closed. I could not have handled seeing her in there anyway. I wanted my most vividly memorable image of her to be from her life. The cremation was delayed for reasons never clearly explained to me, a very discomforting development. The burial of the ashes took place when we returned from our initial mourning period with *Kathie's* family in St. Louis.

The funeral

The small room was sparsely populated with friends and family. Most of the family was unable to come in from thousands of miles away. This close-knit family was not very close to *Kathie*. There was geographical distance, philosophical differences, and years of taking for granted that there would be plenty of time to cultivate closeness. Well, we know how it turned out, and the family learned from that. We are all much closer now, and very supportive of each other, and we have learned not to take anything for granted.

The rapidity of the death caught me by surprise and my inexperience with this sort of thing made it difficult to hunt down most of her new friends. Also, no one knew that she was ill, so it was a shock to everyone. *Kathie* was a private person and maintained a very small circle of friends. She was not very good at cordial relationships, and somewhat of a loner. Still, it was disappointing that only a few of her Buddhist friends came to the funeral. We were very new in California, and most of her friends in the Washington, D.C. area could not come. So there was a smattering of friends, including the principal of Robyn's school, who had personally driven her home from school during the last days.

During the seating, *Kathie's* brother and sister had a very minor sibling rivalry moment. I felt as if *Kathie* was tuned in, through me, and was chuckling at this display.

My brother-in-law officiated and delivered an honest and amazingly controlled eulogy. I wanted to say something and I felt like I should, but I was too emotional to speak. Ron was truthful and called it as he saw it, accentuating her good points and acknowledging her human points. She hated insincerity and would have abhorred a eulogy full of platitudes and untrue statements.

At the end, I stayed for a few minutes and cried next to the coffin. I wanted to be close to her, even though I really did not feel that she was in there, just her body. But it was her body, so it was the tangible part of her, not the part of her that made her who she was, but the only thing I could briefly hang on to in this world. Crying hard, I wiped my tears on the coffin, to be closer to her, merging my molecules with hers, not that we hadn't done that more significantly for twenty-two years!

My stepfather drove home. I was in a fog, with no memory of any events after that drive, until many hours later, in St. Louis.

Forgetting

I remember the days in the hospital and the drive home in vivid detail. But I do not remember getting out of the car, going into my house and greeting the people there. My memory is blank until the funeral and then I'm blank again until around dinnertime the next day, in St. Louis. My subconscious mind probably erased these memories because of my degree of pain. I was both hurting and numb at the same time. Physically, I was on automatic pilot. I was alert and not medicated, but not all there.

This typical numbness is why the death anniversary, the holidays and the birthdays hurt so much the second year. By then, the numbness wears off and you are aware, hyper-alert, and a target for reality and sadness.

Remembering

I spent an abundance of time thinking about *Kathie*, much of it in bed at first, pretending to hold her hand or remembering some of her words and actions during our twenty-two years together. This was both a comfort and a torment. The hand holding fantasy stopped when I found enough strength to think about my recovery. I saw that this fantasy had become more of a hindrance than a help for me on my journey back to the functioning world.

What did the children remember about their mom? Ellie was just twelve and Robyn was just five. Their memories were not as numerous as mine, so I told stories about their mom and encouraging them to talk about what they remembered. I continue this practice today. They both retained more memories than I had expected. In fact, they both remembered events that I had forgotten, and not only fond moments. Punishments and arguments were remembered by the children, but not with anger. We particularly enjoyed talking about *Kathie's* habits. Her brothers and sisters also take special glee when discussing her idiosyncrasies. They liked the way her nose would become smudged on Sunday when she sniffed the newspaper as she read it. She constantly rattled the paper between her fingers, producing a crackling sound, which I always liked. She stopped sniffing the newspaper when we moved to California because the paper used by the Los Angeles Times doesn't smell very good.

We remembered the special way she used to roll her eyes. She had an occasional childlike tendency to put the word "sloppy" at the end of normal words. For instance, the name Sarasota became Sarasloppy. And many other things. It was important to keep her memory alive inside us.

Old events, newly remembered, are triggered from time to time, with head-shakers, events strange and funny, things she used to say, and annoyances, which are no longer annoying but endearing in the retelling. When we talk about these memories, I always fill in the details as fully as possible, so that the children will have a fuller picture of her, including the funny, the silly, the angry, and the human.

Passing the energy

I have healthy skepticism about life after death, reincarnation and ghosts. However, as I was holding *Kathie's* hand during the moment of death, something happened that I cannot explain to my complete satisfaction. I experienced something that felt like the passing on or sharing of an unfamiliar form of energy, with an implied message of continuity. If there is anything that I believe, it is that we are creatures of matter and energy. Something makes us aware. This energy could be called the soul, or whatever. We know from physics that energy cannot be destroyed, including our own energy. Energy can move or change, but it lives on in some form. Upon hugging my girls, it distinctly felt like this force was shared between the three of us. Later, I noticed that some of our gestures, phrases, likes, and dislikes were subtly changed and were more like *Kathie's* than before her death. This can be explained many ways, of course. But it does make me wonder.

This is something that many people find a bit esoteric. The electrical current in the brain can be measured. We cannot know where this energy goes when a person dies any more than we know where the soul comes from or where it goes.

My experience while holding *Kathie's* hand for the last time, as her life was ending, and until the moment of her death, can be explained, defined, or rationalized several ways, even though the use of concrete verbal images can be a challenge. The physical sensation started at my fingertips and radiated up my arm and into my chest. I was not aware of any sensation in my head. I felt a sort of warmth and a "quickening." Rather than exhilaration, it felt like an "adding to." It felt like *Kathie's* energy or life force was passing into me.

This feeling could be rationalized as a subconscious reaching out to embrace and hold on to whatever I could of *Kathie*. My analytical nature believes that. But my preferred explanation is literal, the way my intuition strongly suggests. I prefer to think that her energy passed into me, not like a reincarnation, but more of a joining. There are other explanations and it may even be a combination of several things, even though the absolute truth can never really be known.

There are a few examples of changes that feel even more like a joining. I did not consciously set out to change my ways, even though my self-definition was tenuous. I began to study religion, which *Kathie* had been doing for several years. My study of religions of the world had started in high school, and began to wane around the age of twenty-four. I studied *Kathie's* Buddhism when she began her practice, but I never reached deeply into the ideas. Many people turn toward religion after such a profound loss, so this in itself is not remarkable.

A small number of her phrases, such as "speaking of which," which I still don't quite understand, and certain word pronunciations, now with a light touch of a mid-western accent, became part of my communication for a few months. I began to like some things that *Kathie* liked, which I had previously disliked, such as the religious study. Some of my facial and body movements started to remind me of her. All of this is psychologically explainable, of course. These interests provided a familiar link, much the same as how I felt about our bickering. We bickered often, and it was annoying, but after she died I would have loved to return to the bickering. After all, it was part of her and part of us, and I couldn't find "us" anywhere. "Us" was a major part of my self-definition.

The same thing began to happen to the children, including word pronunciations, phrases never used before and a few subtle but noticeable and surprising traits.

I have always had strong ESP. Not everyone believes in ESP, so I am not going to get into a whole ESP discussion, nor recount my experiences. *Kathie* and I did many ESP experiments together. They did not always work, but most of the time they did. The energy could have something to do with that. Or it might just be a way to fill a void, a way to try to get closer to her. We'll never know for sure.

The Mourning Period

I was tired of the helplessness and I was numb to all but pain. It was as if this unwelcome pain was part of my new identity. While in St. Louis, I was truly cocooned by my family. To an extent, I had been a loner all my life. At this time, I needed support and wanted to have someone around me all the time.

Kathie's family gathered together, saying prayers celebrating life, eating, remembering, crying, and sometimes laughing.

The family pointed me in the right direction, as if I was an automaton, functioning, but not on the higher brain level. I was a walking no-brainer, numb but aware that my subconscious was undergoing an intense trauma, the extent of which I was denying. We were all mainly trying to be human and strong. The behavior of the family was exceptionally kind and sensitive. They were hurting also, so the kindness was reciprocated. We were truly supporting each other.

People brought lots of food but I don't remember any of it.

We were in St. Louis for four days. I remember only a very few bits. My father-in-law, quietly purchased business class seats for our return to Los Angeles, so that we would be as comfortable as possible.

Chapter 4: AFTER

Burial

Even though I accepted cremation a long time ago, I faced *Kathie's* cremation with trepidation. I knew that the family would have a problem with this procedure, but it was her clear wish, and I was determined to carry it out. Cremation is not a very big issue with me because I believe that the person is no longer in the body. I feel that the body at that point is a shell. A very significant shell, of course.

The burial was done solemnly; an affectionate and respectful remembrance of *Kathie* and what she brought to us. Ellie and I were alone on the hill overlooking the San Gabriel Valley. The sun seemed particularly intense. The rest of the family could not be with us because of timing, emotional, religious, and geographical reasons. More support would have been gladly accepted, but I had not stressed the need.

The burial was almost two weeks after *Kathie's* death. Robyn was in school. *Kathie* was buried on a beautiful hill overlooking city lights, mountains, stars and the freeway. Ellie and I lowered the box containing *Kathie's* ashes into the ground and covered it with dirt and tears. The box was so light and delicate! I remembered what *Kathie* had said to me in the hospital: life's process was taking place. This strange and sad moment temporarily focused my thinking, which had been very fragmented in my grieving state, making me only partly present for anything.

We handled it well. We cried and then composed ourselves for a somber drive home. I had been concerned about my ability to safely handle this drive. I was surprised at my ability to marshal my strength, but especially with Ellie in the car, I was even more strongly motivated to come to reality, if only for the drive home.

I did have conflicting thoughts about the process subsequent to *Kathie's* burial and cremation. These are questions that many people have but are disinclined to express out loud, and even reluctant to ponder. This may sound coarse, but it is an honest, emotionally charged issue.

The cremation had been delayed for reasons that are still unclear to me. The crematorium said it was an over-population delay, as if the people were on back-order. This is possible, but with some of the media ramblings about these things, questions remained about what was really happening. I felt uneasy about her body remaining in the refrigerated vault for many days, and also about what the family, already uncomfortable about my insistence on carrying out *Kathie's* burial plans, might think about this situation. I kept the details silent for a long time.

I had other concerns. What exactly was happening to *Kathie* during the two weeks between the funeral and the cremation and burial? The mortuary made another mistake by not giving us an option for an urn, but it didn't matter in the final analysis. The ashes were light in the box, which was wrapped tastefully. The box, with its respectful "gift" wrap, felt strange. But what happened to her gold teeth? It makes me uneasy that any mortician could remove gold teeth and we would never know, even though I would not want them for myself. This is one of those mysteries best left unsolved. And I couldn't bring myself to ask a question that feels so petty. A reliable answer would probably be illusive. And I couldn't help but wonder if her rather elaborate casket had been placed back in stock, or if it had actually been burned with her body, as is dictated by law. Dwelling on this would serve no useful purpose.

Finally, with *Kathie's* body staying there for two weeks, how can we be sure she is in that box? Who is in there? Does it matter? I have said that I don't believe that "she" is in there, but it is still her mortal remains, and it would be comforting to know if that were really her body. No, I don't have total confidence in the system or my feelings about the system. But I still feel her presence. I have clarity about her memory and about who and where she really was and is, and that is enough. It has to be.

I hardly ever visit the grave. She is not in there. She exists within the children and myself. However, there is a lure, a feeling of continuity. When I visit Kathie's grave, I always cry, of course, and I visit other graves of husbands and wives of people in my support group. My new Kathy's first husband, Sandy, is nearby.

Then, and years later, the girls' questions and my own questions still remind me of the uncertainty of death, dealing with the unknown, and the nitty-gritty of dying. Kathy also fielded innocent questions from the boys about Sandy, lying in the coffin and in the dirt. It is difficult to talk about such difficult and sometimes gross matters. We all think about these questions on some level, whether conscious or not. I have found that talking about the issues helps, even though these are often matters without real answers.

Loneliness and isolation

During the course of Kathie's illness, I experienced many manifestations of loneliness. In business matters I was accustomed to being my own support. But this new, personal, and devastating world of widowhood was uncharted territory. I did not know how to buttress myself.

Driving to and from the hospital during the illness is a state of loneliness all unto itself. Oddly, even though I was painfully alone on the last trip after she died, I felt as if she were in the car with me. I was in a state of shock, crying, with a cacophony of emotions, questions, insecurities, and I was just beginning to feel the loneliness that would be my unwanted but constant companion until I recovered my strength.

Physical and psychological isolation is part of the loneliness. After diagnosis of the recurrence, despite her desperate state I was not able to find support for either of us because of Kathie's admonition, generating the first hints of loneliness and isolation. After Kathie died and all the relatives went home, my bedroom was very empty and my prospects for a positive or productive future were quite remote.

Brief respites came with the help of my friends and my children. Some of the family kept in touch as well. The support group helped greatly, because there were people in the group who I could call and who called me, both to offer support and to receive it from me. I found it as helpful to give as receive. Both gave me a feeling of belonging, sharing, and support.

For many months I constantly thought of my situation and *Kathie*. It was amazing to me that these thoughts were so pervasive in my life, but it was the underlying current all the time. I had lost my best friend.

I am told that grieving resembles clinical depression, but it differs because it is considered temporary rather than a systemic or chronic manifestation. The length of time started to feel rather long to me, but I never considered suicide even at my most desperate time. At the beginning I lost weight and my sense of humor, but each returned to normal as my recovery progressed.

Robyn was five. She had been very close to her mother, and was a very needy child. I had a very difficult choice to make. She was so lonely at night that she wanted to stay in a twin bed that was then next to my bed. Psychologists are generally against this practice, but many people do it to some extent. I allowed this for a while because I felt it was needed and I saw that it helped. I saw that it was comforting to me too, but I was wary of that. It was not right to put the burden of my recovery upon the children, whether they recognized it or not. The separate bed helped us keep some distance. But I did not allow it for very long. We talked about it and stopped the practice soon. I always slept with my door open, so the children knew that they could reach me easily if needed.

The empty

That just about sums up most aspects of my life at that point. I came home to an empty house. Yes, the three of us were there. But there was an emptiness, so pronounced that could be felt, even molded into shapes. The better part of me was gone; the person with whom I shared my bedroom was gone; my emotional counselor and confidant was gone.

The closet, still full of her things, was worse than empty. It was a particularly intense area of sadness. I could barely go in there to choose a sweater for myself, or get a pair of shoes. I found myself smelling the clothing, most of which were clean, trying to get closer to her. I was desperate. I searched her pockets thoroughly for any reminder, yielding very few mementos. *Kathie* was fastidious and would not have left her pockets full, especially in clean clothes.

There was such finality in the thought of emptying her part of the closet and disposing of her effects, such sadness, and such reality. I would have to deal with that issue soon, and then the house would take on a whole new dimension of emptiness. There would be a small amount of relief knowing that I would eventually be able to enter the closet without crying.

Reality was okay only as a theory. I was still in my own sort of denial, not coming to grips with the finality of the situation, as I tried to fantasize her return from the dead.

I spent time working out scenarios that would bring her back to me. My thoughts were in a very strange state, mixing the impossible with the "what if." I never came up with a workable plan to bring her back of course, so I settled into a reality/fantasy combination during my private moments.

I have a very tactile imagination. During those early days, as I lay in bed pretending to hold *Kathie's* hand, I could remember the feel of her hand very clearly. I quickly became aware that this was not contributing to my progress, and was actually accentuating the emptiness.

It was the beginning of the academic year, so we settled into the school routine, and then the empty *really* hit. I was devoid of energy, without motivation, and without any optimism that there would be recovery from this condition. Many days during the first few weeks, I had only enough energy to get the children off to school and right back into bed to sleep. I knew that sleep was a common way by which people avoid pain. But, feeling old for the first time in my life, I wondered if I would ever find my old boundless energy. I am glad to say, even though it is more than a decade later, I feel younger now than in those dark days, and I have my energy back. I started to regain the energy very slowly, around the second month.

A significant peripheral loss

Cookie, our dog, a six-year-old boxer, was dying of cancer. She died about six months after *Kathie*. I tried to keep Cookie alive for the children, so they would have a little time to heal between deaths, but all of the chemo (yes, chemo) and money (no animal health insurance) had no effect. When she became desperately sick, which happened quickly, I drove her to the vet to be put to sleep. I cried very heavily, but I quickly put that into perspective. As sad as it was, like a member of the family dying, it was much less when compared to *Kathie's* illness and death. I mourned for Cookie, as did my children. But we were so actively mourning for *Kathie,* that it really did not have the terrible effect that I thought it would have. The attention was clearly on *Kathie* and our survival in those early days.

The gifts

Sometimes we receive gifts from unexpected places and in strange ways. It's can be difficult to see them as gifts when they happen, or even upon reflection. *Kathie's* passing opened me up emotionally. I feel that crying is not macho, nor sissy. It's a healthy human release and expression. Yes, it can be over done, but so can drinking too much water.

It's hard to imagine how anything positive can come out of something so tragic, unnecessary, sad, and maddening. But it can happen. It can take time to see the positive things because of the overriding emotional turmoil and desperation. But it's there.

How do we recognize the positive moments that come out of the blue? How can they be called gifts?

A gift is something that is given selflessly, if it is pure. It is something that teaches, enriches, lasts in your memory, and changes your life, even if on a small scale.

As subtle as they might have been, these particular gifts communicated something positive at a time when it was most needed. I am a fairly optimistic and curious person by nature, which helped me recognize and appreciate these moments. I don't think they were messages from beyond. Not this time, anyway.

Kathie came to accept this as part of the process of life. She knew that we were born to live as fully as possible and that ultimately we die, and with effort we can choose not to give in to the pain or allow the process to define our life.

She knew that she could win if she fought hard, even if only for a while, and she acknowledged that the quality of life took on a new level of importance when quantity became threatened. She took each stage with a matter of fact attitude. "It's here, so we fight and win." There was dignity, incredible courage, and single-minded spunk. Her strength and her attitude to live as fully as possible rather than dwell on the dying process not only added to her life quality, but to those around her. It probably extended her life and taught us how to deal with a life-threatening illness instead of the illness dealing with us.

The circumstances taught me how to cry. As sad as that is, the return of the ability to cry is a great gift.

She died with great dignity and love. Her last words were a lesson preserving dignity in the face of death, and how to comfort your loved ones. She also did something during those final days that seemed subtle at the time, but it gains strength as it is retold years later. She refused to go on the respirator. This did two things. It eliminated the artificial prolonging of life, which in this case would have placed her in a helpless and painful state, but it also shortened the dying process, which was better for her level of discomfort, both physical and psychological, and better for the family. This was no death wish. It was a dignified, sensible, quality of life, courageous decision.

When someone dies, people say that the person "lost the battle." *Kathie* spent almost five years with diagnosed cancer. She was physically and intellectually active and remained a good mother regardless of her level of strength. She *won* the battle. The war ends, ultimately, because no one lives forever. She did not let cancer ruin her individuality, her strength of character, or her capacity for love. She carried on with optimism and depth. She *won* the battle. She will always have that, and so will we.

These subtle gifts can become an island within the sea of frustration, sadness and futility. I somehow found the ability to recognize them so that I would not squander the gifts from this tragedy.

New definitions

The school year was just starting and I was filling out the legal papers. The marital status choices in 1989 were usually "married, divorced, or single." Apparently, the school system believed that parents of elementary school children do not die, so there was no need for the category of "widowed." I wrote in my own category of widowed. I was not married or divorced and did not consider myself single. Pressing rather hard on the paper, I uttered an expletive in anger, followed by tears. My new Kathy had the same experience.

The bad news is that once I put pen to paper and made that activist statement, I officially recognized myself as a widower. The word, widower, sounded harsh, foreign, and disquieting, but it was undeniably part of my new definition. We need some definitions so we can have a few finite edges to our lives. With a few edges, we can have limits, and then begin to figure out who we are. I wasn't who I used to be, because, as I then realized in yet a new way, the majority of my self-definition was with *Kathie* as a team, sharing experiences together.

Until the moment of her death, I had known myself very well, and was proud of that understanding, even though it had taken many years to come to that. But now I no longer knew myself, which was a very insecure feeling. The definition would come eventually, automatically, but not quickly enough for a person as self-critical as I am. I worked hard seeking this definition. I needed some frame of reference, because I felt like a blob rather than an individual.

The search began. But I wondered how I was going to find that identity. Did I even really want to look? Would I like what I might find? When would be the right time to begin serious re-definition, immediately, or after my emotions calmed down, when I could see things clearer? Was it best to do it alone or with help, and if so, who would be the best people to counsel, so I don't inadvertently receive or give more pain in the process?

The evolved version of myself came eventually. It was a process of introspection, growth, opening up to new concepts, and living life. It was not sudden, like an epiphany. It took several years to really coalesce into "me." Am I better or worse now? Yes, I probably am better or worse! Even if I'm the same, circumstances are so different that the idea of "sameness" is irrelevant. It's a whole new scale. I have accepted it.

My evolution might have been easier or at least quicker if I hadn't over-intellectualized, but I explore and analyze everything. I'm not an intellectual, so what am I doing intellectualizing? I'll try not to analyze that question.

Familiar people, places, events

It is normal to wish to have your world back the way it was, but it can't be. Traditions and familiarities do still exist, however, even though the frame of reference is different. I looked for this in friends, visiting locations where *Kathie* and I had history, and taking part in family activities.

One location associated with *Kathie* was the town of Solvang, a Scandinavian village with shops everywhere, about two hours from our home. We went only once but it was a particularly vivid memory. About three months after *Kathie* died, I visited there for a day and walked the streets, recalling fine details of our day, pretending to hold her hand and really "feeling" it. This sort of activity was symptomatic of being stuck in the past and not being able to move on, but it was too early for me to move on.

Some religious traditions, even if not practiced often, became an area of comfort.

My California friends were few, since I had moved there recently. But those few were loyal and surprisingly comforting. I was lucky that they helped me quickly plan and carry out Robyn's birthday party. It was a happy party and a true celebration of life, even as I reminded myself that *Kathie* was missing all of this.

I seriously considered relocation, but in order to avoid an emotionally based mistake, I decided to wait at least a year. A move could be very disruptive and stressful to us. Now, over ten years later, I am still considering a move north, to better air and a better environment for children, but they are so established in the community, with school, friends, family, and activities, as are Kathy and I, that such a move is difficult.

Personality changes/the supernatural

Of course, there is no definitive pronouncement about whether or not ghosts exist. You either believe, don't believe, or are skeptical about the subject. I am doubtful, leaning strongly toward the non-believer category. However, there are things that sometimes rock a belief system, and make a person think. Even though I was in an emotionally tenuous state after *Kathie* died, I never saw her walking around the house in a mist, nor did I smell her perfume, nor hear her calling me (well, maybe once). She never phoned me and remained quiet on the other end, and I never found that objects moved mysteriously from place to place.

Dreams

A strange thing happened when I was asleep, perhaps a manifestation of that energy transfer that we spoke of earlier, something even stranger, or perhaps merely something mundane. I dream fairly often, in color, and in rather vivid detail. I hear, feel, smell, taste, get exhausted from running, or get exhilarated by swimming or flying. The dreams are rarely remembered clearly or in detail, and the ones that are remembered can rarely be recalled after the space of one day.

I experienced a series of completely life-like, visually clear, vivid, tactile dreams about *Kathie*. Remembering them in great detail was easy, and the dreams remained clearly in my memory. These dreams started two days after her death, and came sporadically until my marriage to Kathy, with none after that, at least so far. The clarity of these dreams was more concrete, clear, and vivid than any dreams previously or since. It's true that my trauma was intense and that anything associated with that trauma would be at a heightened state, but these were exquisitely detailed and complete, with all the senses involved. Certain vitamins and medications can affect dreams, but I was medication free and my vitamins were not the dream-enhancing type, like vitamin B6.

The locations changed, as did the point of view and circumstances. The settings gradually evolved from the most basic life-like places, into more abstract composites of places we had known together. The point of view transformed from the early dreams that were a great comfort to me, to the later dreams that were less comforting. The later dreams presented growing levels of rejection by *Kathie* but were actually in concert with the evolution of my grieving process. Finally, the dreams evolved into my rejecting the notion of her return, as I increasingly accepted what must be, without the fear or implication that we had lost any of our emotional history.

In the first dream, *Kathie* had returned permanently, no longer dead. The setting was our home. She opened the front door and casually entered. I cried intensely and immediately accepted her back. Then we sat down to talk. I was feeling embarrassed. What could we tell our friends and family? How do we explain her return? Friends and family had proffered their help and sympathy, which is not easy to give, and now it would appear that their kind efforts were for naught. What were we going to tell them? The dream then switched to a scene where *Kathie* and I were explaining her reappearance to friends and family. They did not understand and we had to repeat and rephrase several times.

The second dream, about a week later, had the same beginning, with *Kathie* no longer dead. The setting was a generic apartment. The same embarrassment was there. I cried during the dream and also after I woke up. Upon recalling the dream, I felt that even if this were only a dream, the impression was so real that I could settle for this as my relationship with a woman for the rest of my life. A transition had already started. The first dream comforted me. The second comforted me and provided a basis for going on, highlighting a fallacy that my fantasies had considered. That basis was a lesson. Settling for an image rather than a real person is no way to live. I was beginning to see that, but I was not ready to accept it yet.

By the third dream, roughly three weeks after the second, things began to change. Sex came into the picture. I had none in my life at that point, and doubted that I ever would. This was a very tactile dream. Again, *Kathie* entered through the front door, no longer dead. She was physically comforting to me. We discussed the same embarrassing problem that we would have to tell our friends and family, but that was only in the background and was dropped quickly. We became physical, more tender than sexual. It opened me up to the possibility that sex *might* happen again. But to think that it would have to be with a woman other than *Kathie* was very jarring at that time. Again, I woke up crying, with her words ringing in my ears.

Temporarily comforted, I replayed the dreams every day.

Most real-life traumas seem dream-like when they happen. Regardless what our heads tell us, we almost expect to wake up from that dream. We want the trauma to be no more than a bad dream. Those events really happened. But these dreams were different. They were really dreams. Or were they? I distinctly felt like I did not want to awaken from these dreams.

Three dreams followed, in which we casually accepted her

return and then went on to do things together, such as travel activities, rather than dealing with deep thoughts or life lessons. Each of these dreams was full of love and felt like very positive comments on our relationship.

Tough love, when you temporarily hurt someone in order to help them long-term, could sum up the feel of all the dreams that followed.

About a year after her death, after about six vivid dreams, she came through the door and, surprise, had never died. She had walked out on me to sow some wild oats. I was devastated. She had returned, possibly ready to start over. She had traveled, slept with other people, and survived well on her own without my help. I, too, had done some of that, including beginning my sex life without guilt, or so I thought. In the dream, my sadness about her passing, gave way partially to the humiliating realization that she had purposely abandoned me, causing confusion about whether or not to accept her back. I did not experience anger, so I accepted her at the end of the dream.

Two or three more dreams like that evolved in several ways. The settings became more abstract: a dock on a lake, a store, an unidentifiable place. The images were less familiar and life-like, but just as vivid and sensory. She had abandoned me a little more forcefully each time. In the last of these dreams she indicated that she was not sure whether to return to me.

The dreams stopped for about eighteen months, and then, probably about three years after her death, there was a very forceful dream in which she declared that she definitely did not want me back. She had just come for her things, which I had disposed of already.

These dreams parallel my evolution from dependency to normalization. Now we hear from the supernatural agnostic in me: are the dreams examples of coaxing from a hand unseen during waking hours? There are psychics that insist that the dead speak to us in dreams, and that dreams such as these, more lucid than any others, point strongly to this possibility. The realist in me recognizes that trauma leaves a strong impression on your mind as well, and could very probably lead to this type of dream.

The last two dreams came very late, probably about five years after her death. I had met my new Kathy and we were deeply in a relationship. In these dreams, *Kathie* returned after leaving me, never having died, and was collecting her belongings but not thinking of resuming our relationship. This time, I did not want her back, not because of lack of love, but because, even subconsciously. I understood the truth about her physical absence and I understood that even though she did not belong in my concrete life, it did not mean that she was erased from my life.

These metaphorical dreams were an acceptance of the limitations as well as the scope of the memories, and the acceptance that moving on is natural and really what she wanted for me anyway. Also, I had grown and changed over the years and she had not. Nor had she aged. The ironic thought occurred to me: eternal youth, the hard way.

The dreams have been absent since my engagement to Kathy. None of the dreams with *Kathie* included the faces of any other women.

Is this a natural evolution, brought about by a trauma? Does this represent change and healing on my own or does the vividness of the dreams, hint that I had a visitor? My belief system opts for the psychological explanation and my instinct tells me it was more. None of this had a creepy or haunted feel. At first, I really looked forward to the dreams, even trying to make them happen by giving myself suggestions at night. But they happened when they happened. *Kathie* would have said, "Just as death is part of the cycle of life, so is healing."

Bills/Hospitals/Insurance

Hospital, lab and doctor bills came in immediately after *Kathie* died. This not so wonderful side effect is guaranteed to jolt you into the real world, if only temporarily, and guaranteed to add to your anger, frustration, panic, confusion, alienation, and loneliness. It would relieve much stress if the medical professional could temporarily (or permanently) place monetary demands on hold for a newly bereaved person. Money concerns are right at the top of insecurities and fears that newly bereaved people experience. It is often felt, rightly or wrongly, that the doctors failed and may have even contributed to the death. A temporary billing moratorium might also alleviate some of this perception, helping both the patient and the doctor.

The billing departments are too frequently insensitive and too quick to begin threatening tactics. They are businesses, after all, so it is understandable on a certain level. But they should be more sensitive to the shock and trauma that the person is experiencing. That emotional turmoil makes this different than other businesses.

Insurance never seems to cover everything, and never seems to get it right the first time. Resubmission after *their* error can cause finance charges to be placed on your account, which you have to find the time and muster the energy to fight. I was fortunate that most of the illness was covered, which took me to the point where all that was left was anger toward the clerks, apparently trained to show an aggressive attitude and assume the worst. Many people have bills that far outweigh the insurance coverage. They are left with anger and debt, which can reach into the millions. This compounds the tragedy into a complex series of maddening events.

I became quite angry one day when a doctor's stupid and insensitive office staff insisted that my dead wife was still undergoing expensive treatments, and should be billed for those non-existent appointments. All I could think was, "One day they will be in my position and they will be hounded, and their emotional well-being will be compromised. Good." This uncharitable thought was not meant literally, but privately venting the anger in this manner kept me from hitting the wall and breaking my fist, which would cause me to have to see a doctor, generating more bills.

I was luckier than many, but a few medical/financial questions remained until three years after *Kathie's* death, all due to incompetence or bad organization. I wondered if this frustrating and time-consuming ordeal would ever go away. Finally the matters became manageable, but the experience left its own scars.

Milestones

Naturally, some days are better than others. Especially during the first year, anniversaries and holidays can be debilitating. The first occurrence of any holiday is difficult, even if you prepare yourself for it. Some of the milestones catch you by surprise. The biggest surprise came nine months after *Kathie's* death.

Mother's Day was difficult, but I prepared for it, enduring some bad days preceding it. Expecting the worse, I was relieved when the day went fairly well. Then came Father's Day. I never gave it a thought. I didn't think it had anything to do with *Kathie*.

When the day came and my daughters, still ages twelve and five, began to pamper me, it hit me hard. They were working hard to help me. It was an honor to see my children being so thoughtful and sensitive, but it was sad that they had been put in a position where they assumed the added burden of organizing and celebrating Father's Day all by themselves. But I now see that it was also an opportunity for them to do something active and positive toward the healing process, and I loved them all the more for the effort. Of all the holidays, this one hit me the hardest. I can't intellectualize about the many reasons. It took three or four years to work it out. The grieving soul doesn't always know where or when to vent its sadness. Mine really hung on this milestone.

There is a very believable account of a little girl whose father died. She didn't cry at all. They were close, but the girl did not express any emotion. A few years earlier, she and her father had planted an apple tree. They had never taken particularly good care of the tree, but every year it bore a small amount of fruit, which the birds and squirrels usually appropriated. That year, six months after her father's death, she looked up into the tree and saw one apple in pristine condition. The next day when she looked into the tree again, the apple was gone, and nowhere to be found. She completely broke down. She was finally able to vent her frustrations, anger and sadness. And of course, it wasn't about the apple. You never know. For me, it wasn't only about Father's Day.

Disposal of effects

This difficult and cruel but necessary task, is enough to throw anyone into a depression, a rage, a confusion, a bad state to say the least, even when you're young and strong and still building a life. It feels very impersonal and cold to turn the deceased person's personal belongings into the category called "effects," probably a carry-over from the nineteenth century, when you did not speak of such things in public.

You're lucky if you have a friend or relative to help you

dispose of the...items. I was on my own there. Some people wait a long time before they begin. Some people keep certain items. Some keep it all.

People have to approach this individually. The process is emotional, irrational and grim, even though it is somehow gratifying to give keepsakes to people you love. I had mixed feelings when I saw *Kathie's* sister, Deb, wearing *Kathie's* coat. The image took me by surprise. For a moment, the resemblance physically and vocally, took my breath away.

I knew that I needed to perform this task soon, or I would continue to live in the past. I was unable to go into our shared closet without breaking down, and I needed to have unlimited access to my clothes without having to think about the emotional implications.

After gathering her clothing, there were some obvious give-away choices and some good charity choices. Some articles that still had price tags required a decision as to their disposal. For a while, I held on to a few shirts and sweaters that retained her scent. If that faint scent had not faded, had I not progressed in my recovery from grief, had I not met my new Kathy, I might still be sitting in a dark closet, sniffing. Not a pretty sight.

The jewelry went to the children, as did a few coats, sweaters, shirts, and shoes. *Kathie's* clothes from the 1960's, which we had kept for whatever reason, proved to be a bonanza for the girls. I held back a few other articles for them.

Who am I?

We know that men tend to define themselves by their job title. I, then, would be a theatrical producer, writer, actor, director, teacher, janitor, etc. Yes, we wear many hats in this profession. My profession requires concentrated mental and physical attention for long hours, with few vacations. When *Kathie* became ill and after her death, I temporarily dropped my profession to look after her and the children, eliminating the frequent travel away from home. It was a very clear and proper choice that I made without hesitation. So my job title was now grieving widower, Superdad. I was a stranger in a strange land, even taking into account my active parenting prior to *Kathie's* illness.

My crying was beginning to feel tiresome, not that I cried

all the time, but it rudely intruded when I least expected it. One day I became so annoyed by my frequent crying, that I wiped the tears from my right eye and furiously flung them across the room, with an expletive. The absurdity was not lost on me. That moment found its way into my play, *Interruptions*.

It might seem that my energy was okay. I could do exercises. I could throw tears. But no. My energy was gone. I tried several methods to rekindle the fires, even briefly trying Prozac, but that left me practically comatose, the opposite of what I wanted. The solution would have to come from lifestyle and patience. That meant hard emotional work. Some things would come automatically, but the recovery would be my responsibility. My emotional exhaustion delayed this process.

I stayed home too much for the first several weeks. I dragged myself to movies a few times while the children were in school, and for some unknown reason felt guilty doing that. The movies were a semi-diversion, so they had value, but I was not able to separate myself from my condition and concentrate in any meaningful way. I don't remember much about these movies, and I felt even more alone. I recognized that *Kathie's* death was causing me to withdraw from life.

I had to be strong for my children and for myself, definitely in that order. I had no libido in those early months and wondered if I would ever want to again. Probably not, I thought.

It was 9:00 A.M. and my children were at school, kindergarten and junior high. I was very alone now, still inventing my routine. I thought back to before *Kathie's* illness, and my hyperactive life of producing, acting, writing, directing, doing publicity, etc. Did I really do all that stuff before? It seemed remote and impossible to fathom. There was a stranger in the mirror, without confidence, without direction. What type of person am I? What type did I used to be? What type do I want to become? When? How? I was turning forty-five, looking about thirty-five, and in good physical shape. Ok, that's at least a start. I resolved to keep up my physical activity. What were my prospects? Would I do any professional work? My profession demands complete attention or none at all, so could I do that? What were my priorities? What was important to me?

I studied the possibilities and reinvented my prospects

with different criteria. Most importantly, I had to choose between being a very active and involved father to my children who had lost so much when their mother died, or return to the all-consumed professional life. The answer, like all answers in those early days, sounds simple, but it was quite complex in its implementation. It was most important to keep my active relationship with the children, and even to enhance it considerably, even at the risk that I may spoil them a bit. A new professional definition would come in time, hopefully.

I was able to buy some time for this juggling act. I have been lucky enough to have parents who are supportive, including financially, if needed. Also, I have been fortunate in the investment of the monies garnered from my past professional activities.

Religion

At times of crisis, even people who have not been especially religiously observant sometimes take comfort in their faith. I found my religious appreciation evolving for the first time, with an emphasis on the cultural richness and the stimulating, ongoing debate about everything imaginable.

In the past, religious identity was a fact but not a daily factor in my life. I was not very observant. My religious alienation began with the general attitude at my Sunday school, which was very superficial and ethically inept. My own family did not stress religion either.

The family that *Kathie* came from is highly observant. Initially, my unfamiliarity with the customs and rituals left me somewhere in Never Never Land when I was with them. As I developed my own faith, we came closer to a common understanding.

My religious evolution started with some very stimulating university courses. I met with people who offered interpretations, arguments, humor, and interesting disagreements. This stimulated my intellectual curiosity.

New duties and responsibilities

Without a wife to bounce ideas off of, I had to decipher all the parenting issues and act on them alone. *Kathie* had been a very important part of the decision making team. Even if we disagreed, nuances and subtleties would arise, advancing a positive and creative approach to childrearing. I try to think of myself as a sensitive person, but here are some areas where I am empathetic and intuitive but genetically inadequate, such as female adolescence issues. No matter how sensitive I am, and no matter how much I may try, I can never truly be a mother. I received help at some of the crucial times. My older daughter, Ellie, had her first period on the day *Kathie* died. Thank God my sister-in-law, Debbie, was there to help. And thankfully, Ellie was prepared, and it was a relief in view of everything that was going on at the time.

Believe it or not, my own financial picture was an area of blissful ignorance. *Kathie* had an MBA in accounting, and had a very clear picture of our financial picture. My artistic life was enough for me and I hated dealing with money. *Kathie* handled all the investing, bills, insurance, household, furniture buying, you name it. Now it was my job. Previously, I had no knowledge of, nor interest in any of that. I had to learn fast.

The first change was that the furniture buying stopped. *Kathie* was in the first stages of a re-decoration. It was her project and not mine, and I needed that money, due to the circumstances.

Then, after some detective work, I found all of our files and learned about our financial and insurance picture. Things were orderly for the most part. I *probably* found everything, and learned much in a short period of time.

I also learned to become handy around the house. Not that *Kathie* was handy around the house. But it was time for me to take a little patience and logic into the running of the house. Neither quality came naturally. Now I can repair a door, some electrical, furniture, some drywall, screw in a light bulb, and do some sewing (learned that in Boy Scouts), but no hemming. Okay, I might do some hemming, but not particularly well.

Am I normal?

The most obvious first question is: was I ever normal? Getting past that, there was a perceived normalcy built over the years. The *status quo* was eroded by *Kathie's* illness, but much of the appearance of normalcy survived as long as she survived. After her death, not only were things abnormal by my standards, but I didn't even know what to call "normal."

Before all of this happened, I was always a person who

thrived on change. For instance, I was always reinventing ways to advance my company's standings, standards, goals, and scope with new and experimental programs. Also, since college, I had never lived in the same house for more than five years. I understood about not breaking what did not need to be fixed, but I found that prudent "shaking things up" produced good results more often than not. But *Kathie's* death was a catastrophic change, jarring and resoundingly unwelcome. Also, I had to come to grips with the fact that my life had actually achieved *status quo*, which is something I had studiously avoided all my life. I needed to understand that, accept it, and deal with it, in addition to all of the other issues. How could I make this work for me?

I was a walking nightmare for my married friends, a young widow, "stuck" in a grieving mode. A person in that mode tends to repeat himself. A support group is a good place for this venting. The particular sadness that comes with loss of a loved one was the consuming force in my life, after my children. I was not looking forward to the future because I couldn't see how it could ever improve, and seemed to be stuck replaying the past and not letting go.

At first, my sense of humor, instead of its sharp, ever ready state, was largely hidden along with my sex drive and energy. It seemed as if my life was closing in on me and getting narrower with each passing week.

But life is persistent and the inbred stimulus of ambition was a powerful reminder of what could be. I didn't consciously understand, but my ambition nudged me into thinking about the future, rather than only the past. Almost insidiously, things slowly began to change. As time passed and the healing process took root, energy and interests came back to me.

Kathie was so much a part of me that any fear of losing her completely was entirely unfounded. Additionally, she would have insisted that I heal, or else!

I was surprised to recognize that people treated me differently. This was not always a disadvantage, but it always seemed that way.

At a festival or a park or the grocery store I would see couples holding hands or talking and laughing, or even bickering, and long for a return of that in my life. Of course, that is normal. But as much as I wanted marriage again, it absolutely needed to be with the right person. Patience was demanded because of my conviction not to settle for just anyone. *Kathie's* passing was such a tremendous loss, that I felt like I was in a category of my own. Finally I understood that the category didn't matter. Comparisons to other people didn't matter.

Now with the passage of years, I have accepted her loss and my healing. I really had no choice. In a very real sense she is here always, of course not in the way that makes logical sense.

The most difficult lesson about pain

I was not yet truly moving on. I did not understand that moving on did not mean erasing memories, thus distancing myself further from *Kathie*. I felt a vague undercurrent that laughing and enjoying someone else's presence betrayed *Kathie*. My analytical mind understood what was best, but inside my irrational heart, I was not ready to give up the pain, which itself was a kind of bridge to *Kathie*. The silent, unrecognized pain became a strange friend and a subversive justification for inertia and sadness. Okay, that is a pretty good excuse for a while. But even good things can be over done.

This is one of the most difficult and most important concepts for a grieving person to realize. It is difficult to recognize and master this strange emotional pacifier. Allowing this release was hard work and it felt cruel in some ways. A certain type of denial hampered recognition. Not all of the pain would be alleviated, but I did establish a method to transition from this state to recovery.

I didn't need to hold on to the pain in order to be reminded of the good times. *Kathie* and I had some bad times, too. With some effort, they also came back to mind, bringing a human perspective. This helped bring her down from the pedestal to a loving and well-remembered area of the heart. It is not healthy to refuse to move on. But it was quite difficult to take that first step. After that, it was a little easier with each step, until I could see that I wouldn't lose my cherished memories and that I did not need to feel guilty about having a life.

How long does it usually take to recognize that this pain is an unwanted friend? How long does it take to work out the priorities so that you are back on track? Everyone is different. No one can say how long it will take. We need to tune into ourselves and try hard to be honest. The advice that other people outside my grief group offered, without solicitation, would have been more helpful if they had been in my circumstance, which I hope never happens to them. If there is one thing that I did right, it is that I did not let anyone rush me or slow me down, other than myself, of course.

How long did it take me, personally, to recognize pain as my unwanted friend? I think I saw it for the first time when I hit bottom, almost one year after her death. I had a really bad day and reacted with strong, built up emotions. I recognized why the reaction to these essentially mundane occurrences was so potent, and that it was time for me to get serious about recovery. The incident threatened not so much myself, but my bridge to *Kathie*. I had begun to understand that I could keep *Kathie's* love and memory alive, and this connection in tact, in a more appropriate way. I recognized that the pain was more of a negative than a positive.

It took time to put things into perspective. The process was slow. I think it probably took more than two years to completely work out all of the kinks. The changes were subtle and I really didn't recognize each individual component or the exact moment of success.

Now, with the gift of the passage of time, I am comfortable with the limitations and treasures of *Kathie's* memory. She is still a part of me. And at the same time, I am happy in another relationship. That is what she wanted for me, and what I know is best for me and for the children. But I still cherish her. I have not craved her presence, ever since I have accepted that I cannot have her on that basis. I know that she is still with me and will always be with me. No one is betrayed or compromised. Reality is acknowledged, with a little idealism thrown in. And, yes, there is still some pain. There always will be.

There are a few lines in my play, *Interruptions*, that kind of sum up how I felt about the pain and her pain. The Pizza delivery man/angel/healer says to Bob, the widower: "This is a one day at a time proposition. You have faced something that the manual says a young person should not have to face. But you got it. The End. She doesn't deserve what she got, right? Of course she doesn't. Hey, you feel guilty. That you're alive and she's dead. That you can have fun and she's dead. That you can laugh and she can't. It's a bad thing that both of you have faced. Very lousy. You're just suffering from intention deficit disorder."

And then his deceased wife, who has returned temporarily, in order to help him, "You gonna live fatalistically all your life?"

Bob counters with, "You didn't live fatalistically, and you died." He was still holding on to that pain, and still felt that he needed to negate any attempt to console his feelings.

Seeking help

I was in unfamiliar territory, in serious trouble with no support system around me, with the exception of my children. My friends were great but repeating and elaborating my memories and feelings were uncomfortable for them to hear, especially from someone who represented their worst nightmare, a young widower. In other words, I felt as if I no longer had any peers. I was without a safe place where I could pour my heart out whenever I needed to, however frequent.

Help came from many quarters, a bit at a time. There were a few somewhat appropriate books. I groped around, looking for support groups, and sought out psychological help.

A support group seemed like a possible safe haven. I could repeat myself, pour my heart out, and help others, within a peer group that had gone through similar trauma. That makes a big difference. Everyone's level of trauma varies, as do the fine details. No one really understands widowhood unless they have been through it, although they may try. It had been clearly established that my trauma was deep.

The support groups

I had never been in a support group prior to the widow/widower groups but I knew that it was the best thing for me. Before finding the group of young widows and widowers, I tried another group. It was immediately obvious that this experience was not right for me. Not surprisingly, the group consisted of retired folks who had been widowed through a more natural course of time. They were between twenty and fifty years older than I, with some similar and many entirely different problems and priorities. As compassionate as the people were, the communication was not on the same wavelength as it would be in a group with people more my age. When the meeting was over and people were going home, the leader and some of the group members tried to "guilt" me into returning, probably sensing my lack of connection. But no one ever called me, not even the leader, so my decision to stop was easy.

I needed to find a support group for young widows and widowers, but it was difficult to find one in 1989. The American Cancer Society, the Wellness Community, and several religious institutions, had no clue about support groups for young widows. They undoubtedly do now.

Then, about six months into my search, I stumbled into a forum for recently bereaved people, sponsored by Northridge Hospital. They handed out a list of support groups, and it was amazing to see that there was one specifically for young people. It was a non-sectarian group, which met at the Stephen S. Wise Temple in Los Angeles. The group has since grown and branched off to its own private entity called Our House.

There were three groups under this banner. The group that was appropriate for me was for the newly bereaved, for those still unable to imagine any future. The other groups were for those experiencing the transition into dating and thinking more about the future.

Wasting no time, I called early the next day and left a message. After some time, Jo-Ann Lautmann, the leader, returned my call. We had a strange conversation. Over the phone, my first impression of the leader was not good. She sounded a little hard, a little impatient, maybe a little angry, and a little demanding. At the beginning of the conversation she gave me what felt like a hard time but she mellowed into a more friendly tone by the middle of the call. I felt hesitant. Was this going to be a challenging rather than nurturing experience? I decided to give the group at least one shot. My impression of her changed for the better the moment we met face-to-face. Any harshness or challenging manner was orchestrated with sensitivity in order to coax, cajole, nudge, and nurture us into participating in our own recovery.

I joined the group and found people with problems like my

own! I no longer had the perception that I was the only one with my problem. That was an immediate benefit, and an important revelation.

The group was supportive, as distinguished from therapeutic. Everything about the group felt right, except for my reason for being there, of course. The people were warm and understanding; they had been through the same experience, with differing circumstances. The room was small but comfortable and lit with incandescent rather than fluorescent light, giving a very warm and cozy feeling and making it easier to relax, and, easier to "let go," if necessary.

My first contact with the group was at a dinner two hours before the meeting, populated by a few of the veterans who were already doing fairly well. Typical of newly bereaved people, I doubted that I would ever be doing quite as well as these people. Two were smoking, which amazed me, under the circumstances. Many of us are still friendly, with a bond that has survived over time, if diluted with marriages and recovery. The personal connection was heightened by our dinners, which remained routine prior to meetings. During that first dinner, I ordered, watched, and listened. All of this was very new to me and I was nervous. Among other things, I knew that crying was expected from time to time. But crying was still so new to me that I felt ill at ease as my imagination projected the scenario for the evening.

Upon entering the room for the first time, it was clear that I had been right about my need for this support, and that this was the way. I was given a few names of psychiatrists and psychologists that specialized in grief management for young widows and widowers. I was given various hints that turned out to be useful for managing the daily struggle, including information about social security benefits for young widows/widowers with children.

My success with psychology was limited at best. The first psychologist was very judgmental, which squelched me. The second seemed so strange and alienating, that I never could open up. I think that part of the problem was that I was emotionally uncomfortable and carried some resistance to the process of psychology. Many people go to psychologists, with much success, but I still had a barrier and I had not met the one that was right for me.

So psychology did not work for me. In my case, success came from real world grief management. The support group allowed me to meet some of my most important friends, as well as my wife-to-be, so it was successful beyond my wildest dreams. Most people did not meet a husband or wife there, but we made many life-long, trusting friendships.

It is important to understand that the group is support, not psychology. No, it was not perfect. Yes, there were some insensitive things done and said. We promised not to judge anyone, but to accept each other and help each other work through our problems. Sometimes the non-judgmental rule was broken, through human nature, jealousy, or insensitivity. An after-meeting gathering at a coffee house might inadvertently omit some people. The leader or a group member might monopolize the conversation, or say something that might sound unkind. These moments do stand out because of the sensitive nature of the subject matter. I did not expect absolute perfection, but the group turned out to be an incredibly positive, successful experience.

Recovery from grief is hard work. A support group definitely lessens the burden. People say whatever they want, and so I talked about and heard all sorts of horror stories having to do with the legal system, social security, finances, the medical profession, health insurance and hospitals, everyday annoyances, fears of death and life, and our children's ordeals. We shared our pain, whether emotional or physical, and the predicament of coping with all of the adjustments. We could talk about and repeatedly dwell on any issue that seemed important at the time, from daily household chores, to children, to gory details of the death.

The soft lighting, the snacks, and boxes of tissues were comforting. We met for about one and one-half hours every other week. We also had a phone list and we used it often between meetings. Those on the other end of the phone felt good about being available, even if no definitive advice was possible, and it often was not. There is no quick and easy solution to grief and accompanying situations.

I also heard about successes, both small and sizable. We delighted in the positive stories, often laced with ironic humor. One person had a first date after two and one-half years. This was a big step. In this case, it did not lead to a second date because her date's fly was open the whole time and he completely monopolized the conversation by talking about himself and his difficulties with women. He chewed with his mouth open, he tripped going in and coming out of the restaurant, he forgot where he parked his car, and tried to kiss her good night in a very sloppy and aggressive way. It is hard to imagine a worse date, but it was a date, and that was a success for her. Later, she had much better luck and is now married, with a new baby, who also chews with his mouth open.

Other successes included surviving the first anniversary of the death, having a positive discussion with a heretofore unreasonable in-law, having a good time with the children, and more.

And there are laughs in the support group. Among friends, we enjoyed a few oases of humor, sometimes of a gallows nature. Laughter is one of the most healing of all things, and another device that helps put things into perspective. For instance, the members appreciated the good-natured way that I called our support group the club with the weird initiation. That would not sound funny to many people, but in an ironic way, we were able to laugh at ourselves upon occasion. We took ourselves very seriously, but we tried to be careful not to take ourselves so seriously that it became a negative.

We discussed how our spouses died. The circumstances rival the most unbelievable fiction. We heard about sudden death while sleeping (adult SIDS), sudden heart attack at the age of twenty-nine, many manifestations of suicide, murder, sudden death from an insect bite while on vacation, flu deaths, drugs, cancer, ALS, all manner of accidents including automobile, airplane, industrial, drowning while on vacation, and more. There were a few people in the group who were made widows some months before their babies were born. There was even one person who became a widower quite unexpectedly through the death of his wife at childbirth, *prior* to delivering twins.

We reported how the relatives felt and if they blamed the survivor, rightly or wrongly. We discussed decision making, new definitions, grief-heightened day-to-day difficulties, and degrees of sadness. We pondered and analyzed how we were learning to cope and learning to heal and move on with life, while keeping the memory of the deceased person in a proper place in the heart.

This was painful to hear when I was still raw. At first, I was very negative, thinking that I would never heal, and not overly motivated at first. But I soon saw that the support and warmth of my new friends was healing, and that I was also a part of their healing. When I saw that I was becoming a positive force in someone else's recovery, a typical group experience, my recovery was greatly aided.

Among the many issues discussed was one that seemed to have a constant presence. Which is worse for the survivor, a sudden death or a protracted illness? A sudden death eliminates the possibility of the "closure" that can come with an illness, a chance to say goodbye. But a sudden death precludes the protracted suffering that comes with an illness. It was interesting that most people thought that the way in which their spouse died was probably the easier of the two, if such a term can be used. Neither is better or worse, and we all agreed that both ways really stink. But you get what you get. You have to handle whatever is dealt. There are no certain answers to many of the death, dying and grieving questions, but it does help to talk.

This may be a surprise. The most difficult moment in the group meetings came at the beginning of most sessions. Seated in a circle, we went around the room and introduced ourselves by saying our names, the names of our dead spouses, their ages, and how they died. Most people new to the group cried during this and some could not get the words out the first time. It gets easier, but never really easy. Saying the name out loud, and concretely saying that he or she died is hard and shocking. But it is part of putting a realistic view on what transpired, and keeping the dead spouse's memory realistic rather than angelic. That is a major step. This was the first moment that I clearly realized that as difficult as recovery was, it was really up to me to do the work; that nothing was going to be handed to me on a platter. I was going to have to be strong. That was both difficult and good to realize.

We shared memories both good and bad. Memories can help us work out some of our fears and frustrations and they can provide a healthy link and when seen in a realistic light, they can help us put things into perspective. Memories are great communicators, even if they are not as good as the original experience, although they can be even better than the real thing if the person is idealized.

And the passing of years has a strange side effect, which I noticed in my dreams about *Kathie*. The dead spouse will never age. He or she will remain the same age as when they died. If your spouse was older than you, the moment when you touch and then overtake his or her last age is a tricky time. It is confusing, emotional and sometimes creepy.

As soon as a little healing energy came back to me, after I started to benefit from the group, I gradually resumed doing massage, in which I was fully certified, and more gradually got back into receiving the benefits of massage. Several years before, some injuries to my back led me to receive my first massage, which motivated me to learn professional massage. This helped to keep my touring theatre troupe in one piece, and allowed me to spread a little healing to others as well. I became an excellent part-time massage therapist, with physicians, massage therapists, and dancers comprising the majority of my clients. *Kathie* was my best client before and during the illness.

When a spouse dies, one of our losses is *touch*. Massage is no substitute for this type of touch, but the nurturing touch available through a good massage therapist does provide endorphin stimulus, which is as healing as laughter.

However, I did make one mistake. As a massage therapist, even though I never defined it as one of my true professions, it is ethically as well as legally imperative that I have no sexual contact with my client. In a profession as intimate as this, temptations can happen, so that can be difficult. But this rule is essential. I appreciated that my client was vulnerable physically and emotionally while on my table. And a recent widow would be even more so. During a meeting, I innocently and naively offered a free massage by me, or a referral to another massage therapist to anyone in the group who wanted one. One person took me up on it. I now know that it would have been better not to do this because of both of our vulnerabilities. It turned out to be too soon for me to do massage and too soon for her to receive, or at least receive by a fellow support group member. Similar to psychology, there can be a kind of transference, and the more vulnerable the client, the more it is likely to happen and the more you have to be intuitive and observant. I did not see it clearly, partly due to my need, and we ended up having a physical relationship starting a week or two after the massage. At least it did not happen during the massage itself. The time was mutually wrong for emotional ties and this turned out to be more upsetting than positive. We saw this happening and backed off but not before both of us became a little more confused and probably a little embarrassed, although our friendship has endured.

My children also attended support groups given by the same people, and another given free of charge by the HMO, Kaiser Permanente. Anyone knowing HMO's might think that any group that they sponsored could only be terrible, but the groups were wonderful. The leader, Linda Cunningham, is an amazing woman, who like Jo-Ann Lautmann of Our House, should have a halo over her head. The groups at Kaiser had a fixed number of meetings, which is good and bad. I prefer an open-ended approach, but that is not always possible due to the number of people needing these services versus the availability.

The children's issues were many but the one that surprised me the most had to do with their school environment. They were acutely aware that they were now different, and not in a good way. Some of the children at school enjoyed taunting, cajoling, making fun of their loss. This can be true for children who have experienced a divorce as well. The tormenting was exceptionally cruel.

"Your mother never died, dummy."

"She didn't want to be with you anymore."

"I'm glad she died."

"I hope your father dies too, and I might kill him."

"I just heard that your other parent died in a car crash one hour ago."

Some of the mean words were the result of an immature defense system, and were not as sadistic as they sounded, but some felt truly evil. Most of the time when this happened, the children's friends rallied and provided an extraordinary support system. I was impressed with most of the children who were very sensitive, remarkably mature, and kind.

Ellie attended two support groups for teens and Robyn attended one for children. At one children's group, a very strange thing happened. The parents stayed in a separate room while the children attended group. As the parents were getting situated, finding chairs and introducing themselves, a woman came in and announced that she was going to lead a group for us while the children were occupied. She was a staff member who we had met in the orientation, so we knew that she belonged there. But we had not been asked or told about any adult group, and none of us wanted to do that, especially without any warning. But no one wanted to rock the boat, so we formed a circle per her request.

We were asked to talk about our losses, a variety from the loss of a spouse to the loss of a child. Very different issues. The atmosphere was quite morose and we quickly learned from the tone of the leader and from her own sad stories that the focus of the group was going to be her, not our losses. She was thoroughly depressed and negatively manipulative. I saw this immediately, probably due to my experience with my other group, and excused myself from subsequent meetings. Others asked me why I did not attend meeting number two, and I told them. They had recognized that they were painfully uncomfortable and resented the way that such an emotionally charged trap was sprung. Relieved that their instincts were right, they decided to sit out the rest of the unwanted meetings. While we sat in the room together, waiting for our children, we talked about our children, losses, and our lives, and told jokes if we could, perfectly normal conversation for those in a similar state. The leader approached us later and told us how hurt she was (again about her and not us) and accused us of running a support group without a leader, which is not what was happening. So she may have had some other issues as well. Great mix! We were talking, no more, no less. The children, by the way, had a wonderful group, upstairs, with the other leaders. So it was worth it.

The experience with the children's group points out that even though support groups are wonderful, we need to evaluate, preferably before we attend, by talking to past and present members and checking credentials. And we need to be ready. Keep our eyes open. This bad moment was an aberration, and I hope that the person has since learned and adapted into an effective leader. Most groups are very good for the grieving person. Mainly, we go with our instincts. If we feel that it is not right for us, we need to be sure that we have given it a chance to succeed.

I also tried a different kind of group. This one mixed all ages and loss issues, such as widows, parents who lost children, children who lost parents, and people grieving over more esoteric losses such as the loss of childhood and/or parental affection. All of these are important losses, and should be handled carefully, especially since everyone grieves to a different extent and in a different way. The room was large and the lights fluorescent and exceedingly bright. Each of eight meetings began with a lecture/discussion. Then we broke off into small groups and tried to hear ourselves through the cacophony of seventy-five people talking at once, which our group found unsuccessful and alienating. And the monitoring by the leaders was inadequate. We essentially had no leader in a support situation. We had never spoken to each other before. No one knew anything about the process, about what to say or what not to say, and the issues were very diverse. We saw the professionals for a brief few minutes, and they seemed to be only partly tuned into us, as if they were feeling the pressure of "making the rounds" to the different groups. I actually went backward a little with this group.

My involvement with the group at Our House started quietly. I didn't say much at first. By the end of my two-plus years, I was invited to become a substitute co-leader, with a request that I do more. Once I invited Kathy to be my co-facilitator. It was hard to break loose from group as a participant, but it became clear that there had been some real healing for me and it was time to leave, when I became tired of being brought down by other's stories. The revelations by the group members had been a comfort to me, establishing a commonality. I realized that I had reached a point where I was seeing the future more optimistically and that the crying, rather than being something we had in common, began to depress me. I recognized that transition and after very careful consideration, moved on.

Chapter 5:
NANNIES AND BIG SISTERS:

Recovery: Nannies to the rescue

Kathie and I employed a nanny before we moved to California. Julie was Mary Poppins incarnate, the perfect nanny. This smart, talented, energetic, sensitive woman now has three of her own children. She was with us for about two years, living in our house in Maryland during *Kathie's* illness, and really became a member of the family. This was what a nanny should be. I thought most nannies were like Julie. Wrong!

With my burn-out in the months following *Kathie's* death, I needed help with the children. But finding a person who would be an *adult* with *ethics*, turned out to be a tall order. She would need to be a helper, and a stable female role model for the children. This would require more salary than was comfortable due to my diminished income, so I ended up offering more than I could afford but less than many California nannies expected.

Most agencies had no clue about my situation, even after they saw it in writing, assuming that they even read our particulars. Many of the agencies were unethical, clearly advising nannies to only disclose certain things about their past. These nannies were taught how to exaggerate about experience, and some of the agencies were untruthful about the information from the background checks that they *said* they did. They were too often staffed by uninformed, disinterested people-pushers. This differed shockingly from my good experience with the Washington, D.C. agency.

I was a young, single dad, still in a sexually active phase of life. So I strongly stressed that this nanny arrangement would be strictly professional and could never be more, in case anyone was shopping for a husband or sex. Yes, very G-rated. I knew that if I messed up the nanny relationship by getting involved, it could hurt my children. I relied on my instinct and agency information to decide on the right nanny. Unfortunately, unbeknownst to me, my instinct was *not working* in those days, and the information was frequently bogus.

Our first nanny, age 19, was from a small town in the mid-west and suddenly became unusually immature and hopelessly homesick. Nannies are normally self-starters and considered a part of the family. She was devoutly religious, which I considered a plus, but in her case it included intolerance toward any other religion. Soon thereafter, she hit Robyn, then six. She lasted four months. And I should have reported her. The stroke was not hard, but it was wrong.

The second nanny, age twenty-six, who interviewed well and had great references, went after the toast in the toaster with a knife, while it was turned on, in front of the children. One month.

Around this time, I was getting the hint that I was going to have to *learn* how to competently hire nannies.

The third nanny seemed perfect, almost too perfect. She never showed up for work after the interview, and her phone had been disconnected. This was a little scary.

The fourth nanny was a real change and reason to think that my first experience with Julie was not a fluke. She is still a family friend, but she had to terminate after four months in order to take care of her mother in South America, or to get another job for more money. I'm not completely sure which. She was about twenty-six, a very pretty, very smart, Chilean woman, with a great sense of humor, high ethics and great warmth toward my children. The line between the job and myself as a possible husband or relationship was never crossed. When she left she wrote a letter to future nannies about what a good family we were and how I was a complete gentleman with her. I was so glad that she noticed and appreciated that!

Freaked out by the endless succession of women coming in and going out of my children's lives, we started to rethink the nanny situation to try to get along without one. It took lots of reordering of priorities, juggling of commitments, and rethinking my professional prospects. While juggling, the interviews continued.

Nanny five was a doozy. The agency told her to fake her experience and leave out all the bad personal history and behavioral anomalies. They did a good job of fabricating letters of recommendation. I was not told, and the agency knew, that a member of her family had sexually abused her as a child. This knowledge would have presented a multitude of red flags. She revealed this to me after she had been on the job about one week. She was honest when she volunteered information, and as it turns out, quite manipulative, probably inadvertently. She was very cute and in her own way, just as vulnerable as I, and we came very close to breaking my prime directive about not becoming romantically involved with a nanny.

One day before the children came home from school, Mina was telling me about her sad life. I found myself feeling very sorry for her and wanted to be comforting and supportive, caregiver that I am. She was crying, so I did what my instinct told me not to do, but what my compassion told me to do. I hugged her. Her experience with men consisted mostly of those who abused her. I was different. We were both raw and hurting, both needy, both vulnerable. It is hard to imagine a worse scenario for a nanny and a relationship.

So I hugged her. Yes, I made the first move, physically, even though her body language and her eyes were saying, "Hug me!" We found ourselves hanging on for dear life. The hug was a million things more than a simple squeeze. When we drew apart, which was at least a full minute later, we stayed close. We saw the hurt and need in each other's eyes and lingered there a minute, holding hands. Bells and sirens were going off in my mind. The sane person somewhere inside me was saying, "No! Stop! Cease! Don't be stupid." So I stopped.

The next day we found ourselves talking again. Normally, a friendly association with a nanny is very positive, enhancing family communication. But the conversation again turned toward our hurt and we again became sounding boards for each other. We finished the subject and again found ourselves emotionally spent, not actually crying, but on the verge, and exhausted. We hugged again, unquestionably mutually instigated this time.

Another minute. No, this time it was more like two minutes, and the last minute started feeling a little different...

We parted and were standing there face to face. And it was clear what each other was thinking. My alarms were flashing again and my urges were nagging me and driving me crazy. I turned to go and then heard myself say, "What the hell." And with that, we kissed, not platonically and definitely more than comforting. In fact, rather than comforting, it was distinctly discomforting on that instinctive level. I was angry with myself but she was an adult, I was human, and I was hurting. Maybe it would be good for me. No, I didn't believe that, but I tried to believe it. I couldn't un-kiss her and I knew what would probably follow. All my reasoning and intellectual ability came into play in a firm and unshakable decision NOT to pursue a romantic affair.

She was persistent, and that led me to begin to see her problem areas. She was creative about it, even playful. As she was being a fairly good nanny most of the time, during the time the children were home, during school she was a temptress, a smart, funny, cute, appealing imp who wanted to have a real relationship. I am not sure if she really knew what that meant.

Then one day the playfulness became a little too creative. It was about 8:30 A.M. on a Thursday, and I was upstairs, taking a bath, getting ready for some work in Hollywood. I was soaping up and in she strode, very naked and very beautiful. She hopped into the extra large tub with me. Too surprised and turned on to say anything, eventually I said, "I can't do this."

She said, "Unless I'm sleepwalking, you already are." And she began to wash areas I hadn't gotten to yet.

"We can't have sex." I was proud of myself for saying it and angry that I was so doubtful that I was strong enough to carry it out.

"Really?" And she rubbed her breasts against me.

I was really flustered, aroused, intrigued. This was a Penthouse Moment if there ever was one. But it was all wrong. We ended up *very* clean, but we did not have intercourse.

In addition to her obviously stimulating presence, she was intellectually brilliant, also a turn-on. But the brakes were put on any relationship before anyone was hurt, especially the children!

She turned out to be a child emotionally. What I did not

need at that point was the responsibility of another child. I needed a nanny. I let her go. I wasn't mean about it and I also matchmade a perfect boyfriend for her. She lasted four months with us, the magic number.

When I look back at that day with a sigh, I still feel the discomfort I felt then.

I wanted a nanny for the children, not another child to care for, and in most cases, I got the child. I recognized that by now the children had grown older and were showing more maturity than most of the nannies, so we stopped looking. I was working at home and could remain active, and between Ellie and myself, we could be sure that Robyn was never left alone.

The children and I were never comfortable with the idea of a single lady living in our house, so when we finally gave up on the idea of a nanny, we were greatly relieved to see the end of the disappointment and frustration.

The nanny situation was upsetting. But imagine the effect on the girls, and especially Robyn. Which brings us to...

Big Sisters

With the succession of women coming and going, I sought out all resources that could possibly lead to some stabilization and positive female role modeling for the girls. One obvious choice was the Big Sisters of Los Angeles. The Big Brothers organization had been around for a long time and I had heard wonderful success stories. Big Sisters was new to me, but it seemed like a great opportunity, even though I did not know anyone who had been through the program. They were purported to be of the same cloth.

Ellie was already too old to start, but Robyn was the perfect age. The screening process for the Big Sisters included background checks, which show a few things, but not necessarily anything about direct one-to-one contact with a girl. Criminal records were searched and employment was verified. In 1990 the sisters were matched using a very limited, vague and subjective set of guidelines, without the benefit of the six weekly get-acquainted sessions utilized by the Big Brothers.

Robyn desperately needed the affection and counsel of an older woman. To their credit, the organizers immediately and forcefully drew a clear distinction between a Big Sister and a mommy candidate. The father is not allowed any true contact with the Big Sister, to eliminate any blurring of actions or intentions between the two adults. I completely agreed with that.

The organization knew of Robyn's situation and the absolute necessity that Robyn's Big Sister needed to be ethical and stable so that she would not have the pain of a woman entering Robyn's life and abruptly leaving.

The match was made by the organization without any say from us. My perception about people is good, and they needed my help. They eliminated the discovery of chemistry or lack of chemistry between the two people. The organizers possessed an astonishingly inept view of people and their interactions. Had this been handled differently, I would have been able to step in and mediate, and would have saved Robyn more pain. But once the match had been made, I prayed that my instinct was wrong about the choices. She really needed someone so we tried to succeed with what Robyn had been dealt.

Unfortunately, it was necessary to match Robyn twice. Both Big Sisters lasted only a few months until they disappeared without a trace. Both women were insincere and not the slightest bit caring about ethical and emotional considerations. One even bragged to Robyn about bar hopping, men, drinking, and her history of drugs! Neither was enough to be this position. This was obvious to me immediately, even at the first impression. The Big Sisters organization did Robyn a great disservice and truly injured her. She deserved better. She was handled with total incompetence. She is an easy, affectionate, mature child, loved by adults. She has even won awards for community service and citizenship, which shows her strength despite unfortunate circumstances.

I know that they must have successes, but they needed to change their rules and hire people with more maturity and experience, with better intuitive sense and better common sense; people who would pay attention to the situation. Things may be better now, more than ten years later.

My daughters' abandonment by women

Think about it, first my daughters lost their mom, then several nannies, two Big Sisters, and then there's my love life. I was very careful not to introduce them to every woman I met. The fact is, I never dated around. That would have made me feel like a single, which is not within my self-definition. I am a relationship person. There were a few relationships that looked promising, and withstood the test of many dates. When these ended, my daughters must have felt varying degrees of disappointment, frustration, and anger, unless they didn't like that particular woman. I allowed the woman to meet my daughters only after a relationship looked promising. The girls had a great attitude and liked almost all of the women. No, there weren't that many, although it seems like there were, over a space of five years. The girls liked most women who were nice to me.

Many wise people tell us that it is best to form a life-long relationship without regard for the children. Hopefully, the relationship should outlast the children's' exit from the nest. But there was no way I could completely leave them out of the equation. Ironically, the potential for hurting the children made it harder to break up when it was appropriate. But I knew that marrying the wrong woman would hurt the girls more than the discomfort sustained withstanding a breakup with the wrong woman. This was a complicated situation that led me to over-intellectualize and suppress my true instinct sometimes. And sometimes it drove everyone crazy. But I was truly confused both intellectually and emotionally.

At first, I had not yet processed *Kathie's* loss, and still wanted her. Once I really began dating, I did not look for her in the women I dated. The comforts and quality of affection created by twenty-two years together is difficult to overlook.

Chapter 6: DATING

My baggage

I wasn't the only person with baggage, both positive and negative. I needed to figure out what baggage I could accept from a new woman and what might be too much. No prediction could help. I thought I would know it when I saw it. By the time we hit forty, we develop our own funny personality quirks and patterns. It's life. We have children with their strengths and weaknesses. We've been divorced, widowed or never married, all with issues.

Our bodies are not what they were, which might make us self-conscious, even though the odds are we're more comfortable about our sexuality than we used to be, notwithstanding AIDS, herpes and other sexually transmitted diseases.

My children had always been number one on the list of priorities, with *Kathie* occupying a more evolved, shared position of number one. I was definitely number two. When she died, the children became number one through eleven in priority and I was a close twelfth. My profession, which had been number one at one time, and then much lower after my family came on the scene, was practically nonexistent from the time of the onset of *Kathie's* illness through the time after her death. That absence, in its own way, is baggage, especially considering my previously active nature.

My items of baggage included grief itself, a strong daily commitment to my children, career interruptions, my age (real or perceived), and the inevitable manners that had been set and fixed into my behavior. I also possessed a kind of innocence, having been widowed and not divorced, but that was only a perception of innocence and could not stand the test of reality. My widowhood, which was definitely in the baggage category, was actually appealing to many women. Their reasoning was that I was single but not divorced, a proven relationship man, a proven good father and husband, and hurting. This was good news for a woman who wanted to nurture, but bad news for several women, fearing *Kathie's* "ghost," my vulnerability, and the possibility that I might rush into a relationship too quickly, which did happen.

Labels / Am I single?

No! Next chapter.

Ok, a moment of explanation. Not that I want to tilt at any windmills here, but I didn't choose to be single, and *Kathie* and I had a good relationship that would definitely have continued forever. The prospect of dealing with the politics and mechanics of finding a new woman was not appealing, but I needed to find a new woman.

Feeling single would mean to me that I was a bachelor, and that was definitely not true of my view of myself. In my play, *Interruptions*, Bob said, "I'm a widower. It's LIKE married...in the past tense."

Divorced people often do not choose to be in that situation, and they often hate the idea of being "out there." But the type of hurt that widows feel is that the relationship, rather than playing itself out, was ripped away. Many divorced people feel that too, in a different way, but almost all widowed people feel it. The divorced anger is very different than the widowed anger. Even if the relationship was a bad one, most widows feel a loss.

Divorced people have an Ex. That is sometimes a very maddening and painful reminder of a relationship that was not meant to end, but did. For good or bad, Ex is a simplified way of referring to the former spouse, if separated legally. Okay, I don't like labels either, but it especially becomes convenient for people who don't think of their Ex as a person anymore. I did not have an Ex. I was simply a widow...widower...no. When I refer to my wife...my wife who died...my dead wife...my former...nothing really works. I don't think of her negatively and she doesn't deserve an impersonal label. Ok, no label for her. I would accept my own label of widower on the surface, to facilitate communication.

So, in order to get out and meet new people of the opposite sex, I had to come to grips with a new definition with or without a label. Single, no. Widowed, yes. Does this sound a little like I'm playing the role of a martyr? Yes, probably. But that's how I felt. I was hurt and vulnerable. I could easily be hurt again because I didn't know my own mind in the matters of dating and relationship with a new woman. Or at least I *found out* I didn't understand my mind in that area. I went with the flow, but the flow was weird, from my rather staid point of view.

My body. Was I going to be self-conscious about it? Not necessarily, but some of the people of my age are. I should expect some women to possess that insecurity. I would have to be sensitive about that, assuming I ever have sex again!

No compromises. Not that I shouldn't be as flexible as possible, in my set ways, but I resolved never to enter into a relationship with anyone wrong for me. I mostly adhered to that, but I couldn't always tell. The tricky part was my metamorphosis from a married man, to a grieving widower, to a person actively involved in a relationship. Former understandings and beliefs sometimes evolved into something else. A woman who might have seemed right for me at one point, might later turn out to be wrong.

I was rediscovering myself, a very tricky process for everyone involved. Was I such a catch? Ok, I have some good points. Some see a sensitive man with a sense of humor, not bad looking, in good shape, and younger than his years.

Practice dates

Someone in our support group coined the phrase, "practice dates." I wish I could take credit for it. These are sorta, kinda dates, but not really, because we're nervous, and concerned about all of the issues. We're not quite over feeling guilt for wanting to date as well as feeling guilt for waiting so long to date. So we're sorta going out with someone, but just on a platonic basis, of course, to be safe. It's as if we are almost accidentally going somewhere with someone of the opposite sex. It's a somewhat less scary and very cautious first step.

I had a few practice dates with some of the members of my support group, and I can honestly say that these "datelits" helped me transition into a dating mode, after not having dated for twenty-two years. On practice dates, we went to dinner or a movie.

We talked about all sorts of things, but never about sex. We did not hold hands in the theatre. The thought of mutual chemistry was a bit too much to handle.

I was glad to take part in the practice dates, and I was glad when I felt I could graduate to a real date.

The "job interviews"

When I met new women informally, I found myself talking about my widowhood, which fetched the sympathy of the women. I hated that and found myself working against it, not wanting to use my condition and Kathie's tragedy in an opportunistic way. Yes, the women needed to know about my rawness, but it felt like I was inadvertently using this to my advantage. Intellectually, I know that I really wasn't taking unfair advantage but it *felt* that way until I was able to stand back and see a little more clearly.

As a massage therapist, the frame of reference changed. I was always acutely aware of the ethics of my business. It is a very intimate experience, and people can transfer feelings. As a married man with a prime directive, it was easy to conduct myself professionally with a client. Now I was unmarried. I was single...widowed...well, at least not married. That didn't change any of the laws and ethics, however. But I was a good boy. I met a few wonderful women professionally, as clients, but I never dated any of them, or touched them improperly. There were no real temptations, due to the strength of my ethical massage training and practice. Yes, it is an honorable profession if done ethically, and it makes people feel good.

Are you EVER going to try?

Well, it had to happen. After all, I was young, healthy and aside from hurting a lot, there were no counter-indications. EX-CEPT. I had to ask myself why I should have such a good time when my wife was dead? How would *Kathie* take to these women? What type of woman would *Kathie* like? Wait a minute. This was not for *Kathie*. It was for me. I understood that I did look to her for advice all the time when she was alive. EXCEPT. Does this make me selfish? Am I undergoing Midlife Crisis? What is Midlife Crisis under these circumstances and how do we separate that from my grieving/recovery state? Is that even an issue? Will

I be able to have sex? What is sex these days, with AIDS and herpes, and things I never had to deal with before? Will I see *Kathie* every time I'm with a woman? I even had to change gears about the word "woman." The last time I dated in the 1960's, I was dating "girls." How do I shelter my children from my dating fiascoes? What type of woman do I want? What age? What religion? What, what, what?

All of this was answered at once, with unconscious subtlety. My instinct took over and decided to let things "happen." Okay, that really didn't answer most of the questions, and that also brought up other questions, but at least I was moving in a direction. Hopefully, not into trouble.

It was the nineties. I was mourning and probably in Midlife Crisis. So it was the best and worst of times. I was free to explore without cheating but not at all wanting to do it. I was still feeling the loss and longing to return to the way things were, even if in a fantasy. I was susceptible to the trap of confusing emotional neediness with actual love. And conversely, I might wrongly perceive that something is not working because of a negative emotional state that I might be in at the time. I was needy. I would look at certain couples at the mall or at games, or other settings, and long to have those days back. They looked so comfortable in their relationships. Yes, they undoubtedly had problems, but many looked like they had a solid understanding and acceptance of each other.

It was imperative to overcome my guilt if I was ever to have a date, regardless whether the outcome was fun or disaster. Human drives and an understanding about acceptance eventually won that debate.

My only tool was the trial and error process. I observed habits, children, child rearing practices, religious issues, physical issues, personality issues, whether or not they put the top on the toothpaste, and most importantly what their preferred seat in a movie theatre might be. I was never exactly sure what most of that meant nor was I sure what baggage I could cope with, and I also knew well that my baggage was considerable.

I was concerned about what my family would think of my dating. What would they think if I married very soon? Should I just date and enjoy it? As it turns out, my family became concerned because it took so long for me to get married. It did take a while to sort out the transition from a successful twenty-two year relationship to a brand new one.

This was the starting point for the play that I wrote about the process of recovery from grief. The characters in *Interruptions* are composites of many people as well as fictional creations. The dichotomy I was feeling precipitated the initial point of view of the play. This is actually a rewrite of a play that opened in 1986 at the Kennedy Center and toured briefly on the East Coast. The play was originally a comedy about Murphy's Law (whatever can go wrong, will) and was successful with audiences, but I was not satisfied. The updated version obviously is serious, even though there are plenty of laughs, and is related to the first only in as much as the final play rose from the ashes of the original. Most TV shows and movies begin after the loss and pretend that the survivor is immediately okay and ready to take on the world without regret. Not in real life.

So part of me wanted no part of dating and part of me was curious but judgmental about the women, and even more so about myself. The women had to measure up to *Kathie's* quality in some undefined way. Try measuring with an undefined ruler, one with no markings. Very impossible. Also try competing with a ghost. Not easy. Try competing with an idealized notion of who *Kathie* was. Neat trick. So, at first I was probably trying to re-create the perfect *Kathie*. Then after a short while, after I began processing my grief when I realized that *Kathie* wasn't even the perfect *Kathie*, I chose to look for as much difference as possible. Still, when I see infrequent but inevitable glancing similarities in my new Kathy, who is very different than *Kathie*, I smile.

A perfect person. We all want such an indefinable creation. Since I am far from perfect, how would I recognize it? Since I am human and changeable, the definition of perfect might today bear no resemblance to tomorrow's definition. So perfect was out, replaced with wonderful, talented, smart, breathing, or something like that.

Throughout the process of looking for the right relationship, I confronted no issue more confusing than "What do I want." This was broken into two categories: what do I want now, and what do I want five minutes from now? The two answers were usually distinctly different. One reason for the confusion is that I was evolving from "I don't want anyone," to "maybe, but only on certain terms," to "okay, this is the real world, so what's most interesting and comfortable for me?" Eventually, I settled in to the process and rather than choosing, I went with my instinct, when it was working, demolishing several of my criteria.

All of the traits would depend on one thing: that someone would find me attractive and want to spend time with me. My instinct told me that I had a lot to offer, but at first, my insecurity about my definition and just what I could offer, rang out loudly.

The only truly lasting criterion was a warning to always obey my instinct, even if this adherence came with a struggle attached. I was in search of a significant relationship. Each choice was important to me. Going with my instinct typically turns out right and going against my gut feeling is almost always wrong.

Some physical traits appeal more than others, but I really did not want shallow ideals to dictate the rest of my life, so I tried to limit this interference. I did, however, decide early on to be sure that the person was a non-smoker, in good health, and physically active. Facial make-up was never a big deal with me, but I wanted to be with a woman not slovenly nor artificially made-up, but more fresh and natural in appearance.

My early dating guidelines included a feeling that I should stick with women from the east coast, my main frame of reference. My feeling was that east coast women were more deep, sensitive and genuine. Fortunately, this stupid prejudice didn't last.

I wanted a professional woman at first. Later, I was more interested in the number of children and their ages. A woman with money would have been perfectly acceptable, but I never considered it in my list of criteria, and I never met a wealthy woman with whom I had a particular affinity.

Ultimately, the baggage and traits that I wanted in a woman came down to one package: a warm, honest, loving woman.

My relationship-motivated mind suffered considerable culture shock when I took my combined mid-life crisis/mourner's confusion into the "market place." The dating scene had changed a lot since my dating days in the 60's! As had I. It could be gratifying to meet interesting people, learn new things, relearn how to love, and eventually rediscover what sex was all about. I did not want to inadvertently "use" someone badly and hurt her. I wanted to do all of this and graduate no more damaged than I was when I started. That would take some real care.

How would the children accept my dating?

Some children in this situation experience jealousy, betrayal, misplaced anger, and guilt. My children were hungry for female affection and support. I was extremely sensitive and giving in those areas, but I'll never be a woman. Duh. So an additional potential mine field for the children would be a premature bond with a woman who might not end up as their stepmother. The children would be in line to experience another female loss starting with their mom, nannies, big sisters, and now my girlfriends.

I decided to introduce the girls to the women only after I saw that a relationship was ongoing. I would have to be careful not to accidentally imply more about the relationship than was warranted or fair for them to hear. Some people introduce their children to everyone they date. That's unfair to the children. Some hold out until the two people are engaged. That is too secretive for my life style. I was looking for a wife, certainly, but also someone who would be good with the children, so it was important that they meet and interact at some carefully chosen time.

The healthy and proper order of priorities for my new partner would be a wife first, and then a stepmother. I had to fight my emotional desire to place the children first. The children move out of the house soon, so if your relationship doesn't have a strong basis in love, you're doomed once the children exit. With a strong basis in love that does not depend on the children, the children will feel better toward the stepmother and feel less pressure to carry part of the relationship, in most cases. In many cases, it can take quite a bit of adjustment for the children, and sometimes it completely fails.

I was lucky that my children were very accepting about my dating. They liked all but one of the women, and that was a big surprise for me because that woman totally captivated me. Part of that reaction came from the timing. It was too early for them to see me smitten rather than casual. Also, that particular woman was going through a set of conflicts in her love life which probably caused her to be distant to the children, or maybe their instinct told them that either she was not good with children or she was not good for me.

I met women in a variety of settings, including fellow massage therapists, blind dates, support group friends, friends met in a single parent group, and ads.

I tried two groups. One was a "Singles" group, for sure. My first and last meeting with them was a pool party. I brought my youngest daughter and we actually swam and got our hair wet. That singled us out immediately. Being a man, I was in the minority. There were probably twelve women and three men. I usually like those odds, but here it was alienating, intimidating, yet remotely interesting. This was one of those times when I was standing outside of myself, looking down at myself and commenting on what I was seeing and doing, or rather, not doing.

I was definitely more of an observer than a participant. Anger, disappointment, money problems, and frustrations relating to divorce were expressed freely. It is good that there was open communication about troubling matters, but that furthered my discomfort profoundly, being the only widower, and because of that I was different in an uncomfortable way.

I was approached rather aggressively by a few women who immediately sensed my discomfort and could tell that I was not really "there," and dropped me, usually in mid-sentence. I went home that afternoon having learned not to do that again. Fortunately, Robyn enjoyed her swim.

Then, the prospect of a single parents' group more linked with religious traditions, became attractive to me. These people were not hard-core single, although I was still the only widower. They were interested in traditional cultural experiences for their children, as well as some social events with like adults. That was appealing, and the people, for the most part, were very sensitive and genuine. We had a hard time keeping the group together, however, due to the diverse ages of the children. Many of the women were interesting, and I dated two of them for a while, not at the same time.

We often talked about single's issues. As the only widower, many of my experiences were different, but there was some common ground. One of the perpetual issues is always the diffi-

culty of meeting eligible partners. We had fun trying to figure out
creative ways to meet people. There aren't too many creative
ways. But there was one method that got us talking, laughing, and
finally doing something positive: personal ads had come to be one
modus vivendi.

Single's ads

There's a real difference between dating as a teenager in
the 1960's and dating as a mature man in the 1990's. For instance, in the 1990's ads are both a respectable and nerve wrack-
ing way to meet people. Answering and composing ads was an
adventure in itself.

First I had to interpret what to believe about the ads.
What does "comely" really mean? When she says she likes tall
men, does that mean 6'+ or simply taller than she? I know what
zaftig means. "Cute" can have many interpretations, as can
"attractive." What if she hates me? What if I can't talk (not my
usual problem)? What if I can't shut up (that's more like it)?

So I met some women for coffee. The coffee meeting allows
for a mutually available quick get-away if things begin looking like
a Grade B horror movie. During the "coffees," I learned that there
are many desperately lonely people out there, just in need of a big
hug and some compassion, if not passion. It was sad to think of
it, but really, I was one of them. The idea of meeting a woman for
coffee and then not finding enough chemistry to pursue it further,
freaked me out. Rejecting can be just as bad as being rejected,
even on a coffee-only basis.

Chemistry between two people is usually clear right away.
But there are many factors which might cloud the recognition of
true chemistry, such as being "new" at the dating scene, desperate
loneliness, sexual neediness, physical attraction, excessive compliments from the other person, perceived common ground, and
more, including over-intellectualizing this process by spending too
much time analyzing all of these things. So I mainly relied on gut
reaction, my instinct, when it was not clouded by over-intellectualizing.

Sometimes my intuition does not tell me specifically where
it is going. I guess that at those times, my intuition speaks instinc-
tively and I perceive intellectually. When I met Carla, who you

will meet shortly, my instincts told me there was that indefinable chemistry, but that we would not and should not end up together permanently. This was most confusing for me, and I over-intellectualized and muddled the issue.

Meeting women in a neutral corner, like Starbuck's, turned out to be a useful tool. We would talk about our experiences leading up to becoming single. Usually my story won. Then I'd get sympathy, which made me uncomfortable. It felt like I was benefiting from the saddest event in my life. But it truly represented who I was. As the Coffees progressed, the repetition began to feel even more like a job interview.

This felt too much like being a "single guy." This is perfectly right for some, not right for me. Then I would stop trying. Somehow that worked even better, causing me to irrationally feel a little dishonest, even though I was really being brutally truthful. And sometimes I momentarily fell back to feeling a certain misplaced dishonesty toward *Kathie*. In the world of guilt feelings, this felt almost as if I had forgotten that she was gone, almost as if I had forgotten that she was ever there. That was not even remotely true, but guilt can be persistent and illogical.

We would either call each other after the coffee, or not. I never knew who was supposed to call if the woman had arranged the meeting. I must have had over a dozen such coffees in the five years. They are like blind practice dates.

But ads are also scary and full of danger if not handled very carefully. A friend in my support group met a man through an ad. Jon had briefly been in one of the Singles groups and seemed like a nice guy. Anne asked me about him and I told her what I knew, which was not much. They became very serious very quickly. Unfortunately, Jon was poking around, answering ads and preying on women financially, when they were at a vulnerable point in their lives. Anne fell into this trap, but much to her credit, she used the support group in the best possible way. We were not given to being dispassionate observers, so we offered our strong advice, which she acted on before too much harm had been done.

My support group had many interesting, attractive, smart women, but even though I was drawn by our similar situation, I felt it would be a little incestuous to date these women. I eventually did date four women from my group, three of them platonic practice dates. My new Kathy was in another group, so it didn't feel so wrong, especially after waiting almost three years to date her, when we were both out of the group.

During the course of my coffee quest, I met a fascinating variety of women. A woman with bank accounts in the Cayman Islands bragged to me, a complete stranger, about her quasi-legal financial arrangement. We were set to meet at a restaurant and she was late. I only had a general description, so I stopped each single woman who might have fit and asked if they were she. Each time I felt a little smaller. By the time she showed up, I was ready to hide, but toughed it out during a fairly dispassionate and business-like hour. Not the best combination of adjectives for a potential relationship.

One woman had been a nurse/receptionist for one of *Kathie's* doctors, complete with horror stories of how the doctor pursued her, again told to me, a complete stranger. She was very different from the way that she described herself, and her personal hygiene left a little to be desired, especially on a first meeting.

A piano teacher eight inches taller than I, was very interested in pursuing the relationship. She sent me a cute card and phoned me, quite within the realm of proper behavior. She was kind of exotic, talented and funny but my insecurity and conditioning couldn't get over the size difference.

Other new acquaintances included a very interesting and nationally prominent, but troubled, handwriting analyst, two real estate brokers (no, they didn't try to get me to list my house), an advertising executive, and a couple of people I never did figure out. Most were divorced and one had never married. I saw lots of hurt and anger. My goal was a relationship and marriage and most of the women appreciated that. I did not knowingly go with a person dedicated to staying single. Okay for them, but not right for me.

I was completely freaked out by two women who let me know that they were not yet divorced, but were planning to be "sometime soon." And there was a doctor, who would have been interesting if she had a possessed sense of humor. I somehow missed this over the phone. It is not like me to miss these things.

Yes, there is an initial phone interview. It's a little difficult to get started, but it's not as bad as it seems. Or maybe it's worse.

Here is how the process works. I called a newspaper and dictated an ad. Then, like most people, I recorded a greeting on an electronic mailbox with a pin number for response retrieval. This adds more details, and adds a little personal touch. Then I waited. My message did not give my complete name or phone number.

It does present a challenge. In thirty seconds do I tell my complete life story, get very clever, or comment on how strange this whole process is? It varies of course. I told about my baggage and passions in life. Both sides of the coin. It's interesting that my children, who give me the most pleasure and pride, could be associated with the term Baggage. It does disclose that anyone who stays with me has to share me with the children.

Interested people left a first name and phone number. After retrieving the numbers, I then became nervous and pondered whether to make the call. Judging from her voice, what does she look like? From her voice, is she warm and loving? From her voice, is she honest? Well, you can't tell from a voice.

If I did call, it went something like this:

"Hello."

"Hi. This is Gary from the ad in the Journal." Silence. "So, who speaks first?"

Silence.

Awkward laugh.

Then she says, "Which one are you..."

It's more than a little impersonal at first. Once I survived that and began the human interaction, it was better.

The phone interview gets out some of the basics: children, hair, weight, height, religion, politics, sports, foods, or some combination therein.

The other way is to answer an ad. I was never ready for the call from the person who placed the ad and prayed that I'd be out of the house so my machine would answer. I could listen to the voice later, which would have told me nothing, of course. About half the time there was no response from my ad. About one-half of the messages came when I was out. The only ones I did not return were the ones where no phone number was left. Yes, that happens, and if it is your only response from your ad, which it was for me one week, it can drive you crazy.

Luckily, I never knowingly answered an ad from a friend, a relative or an axe murderer. Why answering an ad from a friend would be embarrassing, I don't know, especially since she would have been in the same place as I, but it just felt like it would be terrible.

Ads are as varied as the person behind the ad. Here are two fairly typical ads and one atypical one (NOT my ads!):

PRINCE CHARMING I'm not. I just love life and want to have the perfect partner with whom to share it. I'm 35, 5'11", 165#, into fitness and the arts. Will you be my princess?

YOUNG WIDOW in search of a kind man. I have two talented, beautiful children, ages 12 and 16. Non-smoker, small but full-figured, 40 something. Into cooking, theatre, all sports and hugging. Partial to the beach and the mountains, with a fireplace going.

ASLEEP 100 YEARS. Need a kiss to wake me up. The king's guard will be off duty at noon every day. I can answer the phone, but I may sound tired. Oh, and I'm also a frog. Temporarily.

The phone message is usually straightforward and gives information that would either quickly eliminate the person before any embarrassment, or tell important clues that could lead to a successful commonality. Mine was improvised, but some people script their phone message. It is strange when the message is obviously being haltingly read rather than spoken colloquially. Since I was in the theatrical profession, I was aware that I did not want my message to sound too slick, and conversely, I was overly aware when phone messages that I heard spoken by women sounded crude, and tried hard to overlook that in the assessment of the person. Performance criticism was definitely out of place in this setting. My phone message went a little like this:

> *Hi. I'm Gary. I guess I'll start with the best stuff. I have two beautiful girls and I don't pretend to be objective about them. I love animals and the arts. I cherish sharing with the right person in an honest and giving relationship. I'm a relationship person and my goal is marriage with the right person. I am not interested in dating more than one at a time, so I'm probably a little selective, based on chemistry. I look young for my age and my maturity level ranges from twelve years old to my age. I like the twelve better. I'm looking for an unpretentious woman who can share and accept support as easily as give it. Since I'm short, I gravitate to shorter women. I like to talk and "argue" all sorts of issues. Okay, my time is up. Call me if you want to at XXXX.*

So what have we here? A primal force or something? A subconscious prime directive to be in a relationship?

It is clear that I wanted to find love. But at first I still loved *Kathie* with a desperate immediacy, so how does that fit in? I required a little time to begin the recognition of the evolution in my love for *Kathie*. There is a difference between *loving* and being *in love*. Both fit into the realm of beautiful human perks that our creator gave us. Being *in love*, to me, is more immediate. Both conditions are important but one is a constant condition and the other is an evolving scenario. *Kathie's* death blurred this distinction for a while until I settled into love, appropriate for the real world in which I found myself.

Over the next five years, I acquired a few interesting relationships. Upon recounting them, they seem to be many, but five years is a long time. It is four years longer than I had predicted.

But I got off to a bad start.

I was clueless and really screwed up the first time. Here is a story of how ads can be deceiving and how important it is to keep your defenses up and your eyes open. No, she was not an axe murderer, but there are true dangers out there.

Here is an ad that attracted my attention:

PASADENA BEAUTY. Successful professional in search of perfect soul mate. I am talented, young, beautiful, if that matters, but I enjoy Beethoven, Beach Boys, magic, Richard Pryor, and a little Plato. If you like to talk and laugh and want complete, life-long loyalty and honesty, I'm your girl.

I answered Belinda's ad because it seemed friendly, witty, and the publication is highly regarded. Her voice sounded sweet and she was funny, smart, and well educated, with a very good phone manner. She was a CPA, the head of her own firm. She said she was thirty-five, with long blond hair, tallish, thin, and practically a twin of the actress Linda Evans. I suggested dinner out her way, which was about one hour from my house, on a good day. I listened to REM's latest and best album twice on the way there. I can never hear it now without recalling that night.

I rang the doorbell. She was finishing her make-up, but over the intercom she invited me into the living room. I sat down and scanned the room. She had the place tastefully decorated for the most part, punctuated by tribal masks, which can only be described as faces of death and torture. Was this an omen? Could she have been the model for these masks?

She said, "Okay, here I come," which I should have taken as a warning.

Like Loretta Young in her 1950's TV series, she glided down the stairs...well, more like Morticia from the Adams family. I couldn't help noticing that her description over the phone was a little different from the vision before me. She was a little heavy, not fat, but not thin as she indicated. She looked like she never worked out or exercised at all, rather than the exercise freak that she described. The long blond hair described over the phone had been replaced by medium darkish brown, with obvious gray roots, and Linda Evans was nowhere to be seen. I really don't like to dwell on physical attributes, but she made such a point of the fact that she was gorgeous and young. Here was a woman who was most unattractive and several years my senior. Okay, now how do I get out of this? I really had no useful thoughts in that direction. I am a nice guy, so I didn't want to hurt her, even though she had purposefully deceived me.

We restaurant-hopped until she found one that was comfortable to her. It was about 9:00, with my stomach gurgling loudly. We waited until 10:30 for a seat at this chaotic *Singles* restaurant. Everyone was smoking, so I couldn't breathe. We finally got a very uncomfortable table and we ordered. The inedible food arrived after a long wait, the only taste being salt. She was playing footsie under the table and making faces that were a cartoon version of Mae West. I was sitting there, mad at myself, mad at her, mad that I even had to be dating, mad at the restaurant, hungry, and apprehensive about what else she had in mind.

We drove back to her place for what I could only hope would be the end to an embarrassingly mismatched evening.

She said, "Come inside with me."

"I'm really tired," I said as unappealingly as possible.

She said, as appealingly as possible, "How about next Saturday?"

Now Mr. Nice Guy was going to have to leave Wimp City and be real.

"No, I really don't think we have anything going here."

"We definitely do. Come on in and I'll show you."

"No." Or rather, "Nooooooooooooo."

"I'll call you next week. You'll change your mind."

"We really don't have anything here." And I left...I tried to leave. She had my sweater firmly lodged in her fist.

"You have to kiss me first, then you'll change your mind."

Now here's a challenge. I had never refused a kiss in my life. I didn't know how to do it. Reaching over at arm's length, I gave her a peck on the cheek and with this diversion she released my sweater, enabling my escape.

I felt terrible for how I reacted and how she deceived me. I know that some of my reaction was also general dating shock, but I wondered if this would be as good as dating could ever be.

Now the hard part

As I have said, as an adjunct to my life-long theatrical career, I had been a massage therapist, and also an organizer. I continued organizing a massage complex for a health-oriented convention that met periodically in Los Angeles, San Francisco, San Diego, and New York. This was always a mix of interesting people, time-tested health concerns, and new and exciting finds. It also presented without comment some Snake Oil preparations, not dissimilar from the potions that used to be hawked from horse-drawn wagons in the old days, and some quasi-medical treatments with claims that were impossible to verify. This is one of the reasons why I eventually left. I met Lisa, Satira, and Leslye there within a three-year span.

Through the course of the weekend, we would do over 1000 twenty-minute introductory therapeutic massages with ten therapists working, presenting ten different therapeutic styles at any one time.

Lisa: About thirty, Lisa was blond, very pretty, funny, smart, and a very talented artist. It would seem on the surface that I should stop there and marry her. Well, there's chemistry, emotional availability, professional ambition on her part, and total confusion on mine. It was very early for me. We set out to do a massage trade one Friday evening. Massage therapists do that frequently as a legitimate way to learn and receive a free massage.

We were serious about the trade. When therapists trade, it remains business and we never break the line between the intimacy of massage therapy and the intimacy of sex. Well, let's not say "never." We did a very good trade, both being talented in that area. She was single and unattached, as was I, even though I really hadn't come to grips with that.

Without skipping a beat, we found ourselves making love. I was taken by surprise. Had I time to think about it, I might not have been able to do it. After twenty-two years with one woman, with the emotional scars from her illness and a death, I would have probably experienced performance anxiety or pictured *Kathie's* face on that pillow. But this surprise worked for me. She was playful, talented and very sensitive to my situation. I was a 'project' for her, and my 'virginity' was on her agenda for the night. We lost it very nicely. She was prepared with the necessary items so that there was no disease question (I had nothing). We were so intense that I was sure I was supposed to have a relationship with her, even though there was no chemistry to have a real relationship. After her conquest, her interest in me went away.

I lost my virginity. But it was an accident, or at least a covert operation, so it only counted partial credit. I was still not sure what to do or how, assuming a more deliberate situation might ever materialize.

Satira: About forty-two, an encyclopedia of New Age, with two bright and talented children. This was a new experience for me. Well, at this point, everything was a new experience.

She was the massage therapist for Sting during his Rainforest tour. She knew many exotic styles of therapeutic massage and nurtured me with each one. I was compliant but still in a daze, unable to give much back in those days. Our relationship lasted about three months. She said that she was grooming me to recover from my grief, and fall into a relationship with a much younger woman, and get married. I didn't want to do that yet, especially with a much younger woman.

Satira told me that she was an angel who was sent to guide me through the rough spots for a while. In my belief system, angels are messengers, and are not necessarily from heaven, but usually earth-based, with a few notable exceptions. She and her daughter are significantly featured in Dianne Keaton's movie "Heaven."

Her angelic trance-like moments were a little frightening at times, but benevolent in meaning. We are still friends.

Mary I: This was the woman for which Satira apparently primed me. Mary was, twelve years my junior, never married. We met at a birthday party for Grant, a friend, who would later fall in love with Mina, our last nanny, in an intellectual match made in heaven. During our conversation, Mary complained about a neck ache, so I worked it out. Our physical chemistry became evident to both of us. So Mary and I ended the evening with a hug. Or rather, a HUG.

Not completely emotionally alive yet, I tried hard. Mary was an attorney who was smart, cute, inventive, and playful. Our chemistry was good, which opened me up so that she could bring me to life. I was not sure that I would ever get back to life until then, typical of widows and widowers.

She introduced me to the personal and visual beauty of Bed & Breakfasts and put an entirely *new* meaning to the concept of going to a musical concert by the new age artist, Kitaro. Typical of my relationships, we were pals also. Okay, naughty pals.

Now I felt like I was beginning to get an inkling of the new me, and for the first time I truly realized that it felt good to be with someone. She was good to the children too.

But...she was coming off a long relationship with a man many years her senior. It had been constantly rocky and she was sure that she was better off with me. She fell in love (lust?) with me very quickly, too quickly. As we know, I was not in a quick mode. I knew that she'd end up with him, and that it was appropriate for that to happen, and she did. But she made him work for it. I provided no resistance to her returning to him, somehow causing him to have to work all the harder to win her over.

Then Mary discovered a very high priced New Age organization, which reminded me of a 90's version of encounter groups. The group used conventional brainwashing techniques to make her feel like she had learned something about life and herself. The contradiction was that no one, including the leaders, could clearly explain what anyone learned or how it worked in their life. She decided that she could not be in a relationship with anyone who had not taken the program. This gave her former boyfriend with the opening he needed, so the group had a positive effect after all.

So I got dumped, but in a humane and totally appropriate manner. I did not mourn this loss, since it was clearly time for these things to happen, and continued my quest, still hoping to find the fullest emotional feelings.

Leslye: This is the relationship that was destined to happen and never did. I met Leslye in 1987, immediately upon my relocation to California. I chose her as one of the fifty massage therapists hired in my capacity as organizer for the Whole Life Expo. She is rather small of stature with jet-black hair, beautiful brown eyes, and a very strong energy, which makes her seem imposing, in a good way.

There was a definite mutual chemical reaction on our first meeting. But I was married and even though I was very human, I am very black-and-white about the sacrament of marriage, as well as the commitment and trust of a non-married relationship. So I tried my best to ignore her, and she tried to ignore me for the same reason.

Now, two years later, she had just broken up with a very significant boyfriend and I had been a widower for a year when fate and a little manipulation on my part placed us together again. We had only communicated professionally during this time. But now, we were here, unattached, and still feeling the chemistry.

I had fantasized about her after *Kathie* died, thinking that she was very likely the perfect woman for me, even though I hardly knew her and her complexities, and she hardly knew mine. But she was a good age, perhaps a little young, cute, smart, small, funny, sensual...okay, I'll stop. She reminded me a little of *Kathie*, but I was in denial of that at the time.

Now, at Expo, at the end of a busy day, we found ourselves tired and in need of a quick twenty-minute massage trade. We kept everything G rated, maybe a little PG. The room is very removed from the rest of the Expo and each of fifteen tables is curtained off for complete personal privacy. During the Expo we monitored the ethics of each practitioner.

Leslye and I retired to the cubicle assigned to her. We were organizers, so the rules were made to be interpreted by us. She removed her clothes completely, to my surprise, and got on the table. After all, she knew that I had seen lots of naked people through my life, especially in theatre and massage. Predictably, my libido completely took over my every thought. I did control myself. This was not the proper place to do sexual things. We would need to find a proper place very soon! We finished her back and legs; she was very tense from the day's work and from a headache. Then it was my turn. We kept the massages completely ethical and we did nothing inappropriate. But we did agree that dinner and cuddling was absolutely necessary for the night. At that moment I began to experience cuddling anxiety.

I had led up to this for two years. She seemed the perfect

woman for me, and as if she needed more positive credentials, she was a Tantra instructor. Tantra is the ancient Indian art of breathing deeply and fully experiencing and controlling the sexual experience, to prolong, heighten and strengthen it. So she probably knew it ALL. I knew her well enough to just barely handle the safe sex issue. I really wanted to be with her but I could feel the beads of sweat accumulating. So this could either be the best sexual experience of my life or my worst. Guess which it was.

Starting with a bath to loosen us up a little, we did cuddle but we were both exhausted, and maybe she was experiencing some sort of performance anxiety also. It just didn't happen. But I did enjoy our time together and her warmth. I learned more about her rather complex life and personality, and decided that if I ever got over my fear, I'd love to try again.

Since she lived in Palm Springs and I in Los Angeles, this never happened. I do think about her positively, and I know we would have had a very interesting time together.

Sara: She was three inches taller than I, divorced, with a two-year-old boy. We started tentatively and had fitful chemistry, but lots of laughs. One day, she had a bad conversation on the phone with her Ex and for no reason her verbal abuse spilled over onto me. We realized that it was over for us after her son peed on my shoe. My admirably restrained reaction was less than positive. Really, he should have peed on HER shoe. Maybe I should have peed on her shoe. We dated about a month, so it was no major commitment.

Michelle: This very striking woman had electric green eyes and very long, wavy medium brown hair down to her buttocks. We had met a few years earlier, when *Kathie* was still alive and she tells me that she had envied our family togetherness.

After dating for about a month, she told me that she had another guy with whom she was also interested. He lived in Montana, a mountain man who made occasional visits. I was looking for commitment. I respected her honesty and her constant striving for interesting things in her life. We remain friends now, and see each other at social functions from time to time, always with Kathy by my side.

Stephanie: This points out some of the hoops we jump through in the dating process. We're planning the next fifty years of our life, so we try to make an emotional but careful decision. Well, one out of two ain't bad. Stephanie was an attractive young woman with an appealing kind of innocence about her. This was a blind date set up by a friend. It lasted only through dinner that night because we had absolutely no chemistry. But her daughter! She was an exceptionally cute, mature, vivacious, and magnetic nine year old. I would have loved being her step dad, at least from first impressions. And I was so impressed with her that I even considered giving her mom and me a second try. But it would have been futile, and I knew it. So I'm sure we avoided lots of hurt by not trying.

Stephanie was my only authentic blind date, and I was nervous. But my nerves settled some with her soft, kind manner, and also when I saw that she had a little perspiration under her arms, indicating her own set of nerves. Good. She was human like me.

It makes me sad to see how many desperately lonely people there are in the dating scene. People just want to connect with someone, and that is so hard to do.

Mary II: This was the first bolt of lightning, the first chemistry, the first infatuation, almost two years into *Kathie's* loss. This feeling overcame my grief for a little while. Well, about a week. This was set up by the leader of our support group, who also introduced Kathy to me one week later. We met for dinner and I could feel my heart pounding. We couldn't stop talking and smiling. I didn't sleep that night.

She was in a very high profile family oriented job and she was divorced in a totally friendly way. He had suffered severe physical debilitation and she had stuck with him for years, so there was a similarity with my situation with *Kathie.*

We saw each other four times within the space of a week and a half. We became very passionate but G-rated. Well, PG13. We did not date long enough to get very close to sleeping with each other. She was coming off a long-term romance with a good man who couldn't decide about commitment. I came along when she was on the rebound. Sound familiar? Unlike the situation between Mary and me, it was difficult to accept the inevitable.

She realized her need to try to make it work with her boyfriend and stopped our relationship before it got too heavy, for which I thank her. Now, after a lengthy working through of issues, they are married. Kathy and Mary were soccer moms together before I met either of them. We're all friends now and everyone knows everything, even though there's not much to know.

When we broke up, if that term can be used for such a short time together, I felt intense grief for a while, but that showed me that I was recovering, because my immediate grief for Mary was stronger than my grief for *Kathie*. After a little while, the grief switched back to *Kathie*, but I still took it as a positive indication.

Carla: Sometimes we make mistakes. In relationships, the mistakes can be big. I was not accustomed to making relationship mistakes. I had long since made myself promise that I would not settle for anything that would not clearly improve my life. I was not in a hurry and did not need to be. The right relationship is worth the wait.

I am still figuring out this relationship. I took a lot of flack from many of the people around me for staying in this one for as long as I did. Carla was the only person who I dated through an ad. I'm not positive who placed it. Carla had shoulder-length light brown hair, brown eyes, 5'3", with a figure tending toward the petite. She was a runner and worked out regularly, so the petite was punctuated with a well-defined but subtle musculature. She could easily whip up a very complex recipe and she could make dry wood taste good. And on our bad days, she probably did. I saw Carla as smart, warm, very private, quiet, not very attractive in the usual sense, but with a cute smile which grew in cuteness throughout the relationship, very natural, and very dedicated and cuddly to her children. She would have been a very devoted mother to my girls.

Here was an example of mild chemistry, growing as the relationship progressed. My instinct told me that this was a good relationship to be in but that it would not go the distance. Perhaps I saw that as a challenge, because it almost did.

We had a trusting relationship but I think we both unintentionally held back a little emotionally. Or at least we perceived that the other was holding back. Which usually means that we both were holding back.

There were communication problems at the end, highlighting the communication problems that we had experienced but denied throughout the relationship, and her divorce intruded in a very threatening way. Typical of divorces, her Ex was incredibly angry with her. I'm not sure how angry she was at him, but I believe it was considerable. The magnitude of anger that her Ex showed spawned a revengeful attitude with hurtful, even self-defeating actions. It would be presumptuous of me to analyze it. Suffice to say, each thought the other was at fault. I felt protective toward her until the end, when I was advised that if we got married, I would have to shoulder a never-ending barrage of court appearances, attorneys and attacks from her Ex. Carla expected me to bear the entire financial burden and be in the middle of a mess that was not my mess. I was just coming out of a big enough mess. To go into another, especially one so angry would have been madness. I remembered the promise I made to myself.

At the end, her demeanor changed and she appeared more interested in being taken care of than being in love. I guess that is legitimate, but I wanted love first in priority and I originally thought she did too. But now her every action seemed to put love second.

Once a person was out of her life, they were erased. They ceased to exist. I never understood that. With a nasty divorce, you would certainly want to think of the Ex as little as possible as long as there is intense pain, but that does not negate the good times and the reasons you were together in the first place. She didn't understand why *Kathie* was still a pleasant force in my life. She thought it was time for me to negate her or wipe her out. I do not see it that way. She can be there in a non-threatening way. Our twenty-two years together made me the person that attracted Carla. I sometimes believe that it is difficult for many people to compete with a ghost. Competing with an angry ex-spouse is hard, but it also takes a very special kind of mind-set to cope with an absent person whose memory is cherished. My union with Kathy doesn't have that problem. Since we are both widows, we understand that more easily than some might.

We tried pre-marital counseling, which was completely

against my instinct and my knowledge of relationships. I felt that if we had to receive counseling prior to a marriage commitment, there was little chance that the marriage could hold up.

It was wrong for me to consider a marriage from a relationship that started out this troubled. I knew it and yet couldn't let go. I was unanimously coached to heed the clear signal. I tried to let go, and we'd both have been better off if I had succeeded earlier. This process began to show me the other side of her divorce, raising significant new questions about who started what and who did what, even if there are no real answers.

We ended up with a massive communication breakdown. I think we accused each other of the same things. I know I'm out of her life completely and she appears to be angry. I appreciate the good part of what we had together. Two very different takes on life or relationships. Which is healthier? I think mine is. She thinks hers is.

Kathy and Carla met on several occasions. Kathy was my confidant throughout the difficulties with Carla, but she was very careful never ever to say anything that would encourage a break up. In fact, she usually said things that were helpful to the relationship, especially since Kathy thought that she and I would never date anyway. Carla resented the thought of my seeking counsel from anyone, including my family, but people have to get help somewhere, even if it's no more than blowing off a little steam. Kathy reassured me and comforted me and frequently was able to put things into a form that made it easier to go back to Carla, really acting as both Carla's ally and mine.

Kathy and I never kissed or any of those other comforting things, even when Carla was going through some drastic and sudden changes in the rules of our relationship, which negated me and caused us to part on two occasions. Carla and I had an enriching love life. She stressed the fact that even during the darkest days of her marriage she never denied her husband's lovemaking, and would never do so to ours. But toward the end of the relationship, she put a halt on it. Changing the rules after almost two years can only have a bad effect. We derailed each time she changed the rules. She felt that she was suddenly in conflict with her religious beliefs, but apparently had not been in conflict before. It was obvious punishment for my not speeding into the marriage.

She probably knew subconsciously that we were not right for each other, and reacted without thinking, sabotaging the relationship. It was wrong-headed but not malicious.

It was agreed that prenuptial agreements were needed to protect our children. Prenups are often used as a way to protect assets garnered prior to the marriage. But it can be nasty, almost as if a bad ending to the marriage is assumed, and is now being planned. If such a document is needed, it is best to get it over with early, not at a time near the wedding date. At the end, she gave me an ultimatum from left field that was totally out of line and impossible for me to accept on a personal or financial level.

Actually, as uncomfortable as the prenuptial was, it did let us see each other in a light that would have been shed after the marriage, at a time when it would have been too late. So it had its use. Later, Kathy and I needed to do a prenuptial, and it was a more reasonable process, but still very uncomfortable.

Then I tried to do what Carla taught me to do. I tried very hard to get past it and go on with my life, using the steps that she used with her Ex. I had made some progress, as I reminded myself of my instincts and that we were not the best marriage choice for each other.

The inference that she took, probably out of defensiveness, was that I did not love her as much as she loved me, and she reproached me for that, which hurt me deeply. But that was what I thought about her feelings toward me. So there we are. That's again the communication problem.

People still don't understand what I saw in her. What do we see in people? What did she see in me? We saw something.

Here is the crux of the problem. I was unable to pull the plug when I should have because I cared for her, I did not want to hurt her, and unbeknownst to me, I could not handle separating from a relationship that was growing in commitment through time. It felt too much like losing another wife. I was dealing with separation anxiety, which led me to stay in a relationship that was clearly not right.

What the heck was I doing?

Chapter 7: KATHY

I met Kathy Smith on December 18, 1991, eight days after my first *Kathie's* birthday. I now think of this day as my re-birthday. I was at the time newly smitten with Mary #1 and I had just met Carla. But I noticed Kathy. Is this confusing?

We met at an informal mixer after I had been in the group for two years. The leader, Jo-Ann, mixed the old guard, my peers and myself, with the new members and arranged us in groups of six. I know that Jo-Ann, in her infinite wisdom and optimistic frame of mind, had newcomer Kathy and me in mind for matchmaking. It took three years, but her plan eventually worked.

I had an immediate attraction to Kathy but it was too early to date her, although Kathy says she does not believe that it would have been too early. She was very recently bereaved, about three months, and I was too much into the search for a lasting relationship to chance a transitional relationship with her, especially since I felt that she was emotionally vulnerable at that time. I've been there.

Even as a new widow, there was radiance about her, a magnetic force. Her many friends have felt this. She maintains a large circle of friends who confide in her, respect her loyalty and enjoy her presence, her sense of humor, and her natural curiosity. She is a great conversationalist and knows all of the right questions to ask, and you know that she really wants to hear the answer. One person was joking and said that a conversation with her is like an interview.

She was, and still is pretty great looking with longish dark hair, not dyed, and radiantly beautiful eyes. The eyes are almost copies of mine, but on her they shine brilliantly. She is into makeup and really knows how to apply it tastefully and in a way that naturally accentuates her face. Then there is her smile. She has the biggest, brightest smile. It's like her whole face is smiling. When she smiles, and it is often, fortunately, you can't help but smile back, and you want to take her and kiss her, or at least I do. Circumstances did not allow me to do that when we first met, but I am making up for it now. She has a very cute, well-proportioned figure. And she is tallish, from my point of view, that is. She is among the tallest of the women in my life. She is actually considered petite, but at a little over 5'3" we fit perfectly, and there's just enough of me left over so she can wear heals without being taller.

I was among friends at this meeting because I had been in the group for a long time. Kathy was among the group of new arrivals. It turns out that at this unusual meeting, it was very hard for the new people to mingle with the veterans. We tried to be kind and helpful, but the evening was overwhelming for many of the new people. It is hard for a newly bereaved person to imagine normalcy, interaction with the opposite sex, laughter, and looking toward a future with the possibility of happiness. It was confusing and jarring to many of the new members to see bereaved people behaving like normal people.

I was sitting next to a close friend. She had a headache, so at the beginning of the meeting I put my massage training into practice and informally rubbed the back of her neck with my right hand. Kathy tells me that I made a strong impression with that. I was not even aware that it was noticed by anyone. It looked like the woman and I were an "item." We were not. I can now see how such an innocent action in that setting could be misinterpreted. I saw it as nurturing, but others may have seen it differently. I wonder how jarring that might have been to the other newly bereaved people.

My interest started immediately when Kathy and I met. I listened to the details about her husband's death, and the fact that she had three boys. I went on to talk to others in our group of six, but always looked back at her. Chemistry is a very strong thing, hard to ignore.

Within a few weeks we found ourselves together in a children's support group. The adults met informally in the room usually used for our support groups and the children met in another room. One of her sons was running amuck, so I was getting further insight into what I thought I could not handle, conditioned by my previously quiet life. But Kathy and I became pals.

The leader wanted us to use the fluorescent rather than the incandescent lights in our room. I hate fluorescent, and there was a choice. The room was warm and friendly with the incandescent, and cold and uninviting with the fluorescent. This was very important to people who were accustomed to the room in the warm mode, and who needed the coziness for emotional reasons. The leader changed the lights to fluorescent. When she left, I changed the lights back to incandescent. She came back, changed the lights back to fluorescent, and we discussed the situation. Boy, did we discuss it! She never gave me a reason and I gave her three. So when she left, I changed the lights again. One more exchange and she saw by my face that I was not going to give in, and that everyone was agreeing with me. We ultimately won that argument after appealing to her higher-ups. We were going through enough without having to deal with insensitivity from a leader of a support group. My instincts about this particular leader never changed, and were further reinforced by the reports of others who suffered from her insensitivity. And yet she did have her positive effect on the group. Okay, it's no big deal, but the absurdity of the situation left Kathy and me even closer friends.

That step forward led to a moment that should have been another step forward, but not only was it a big step backwards for us, it even became a short term slide for my grief process. One day I came home and checked the messages on my answering machine. Kathy had left a message about a support group function. The message began with a very upbeat voice saying, "Hi Gary, it's Kathy..." That's all I heard the first time I played it. I had an immediate reaction. I burst into tears, hard, and found myself on the floor. I just was not ready to hear that name juxtaposed with my name. Rather than comforting, this message from a woman with the same name as my dead spouse took me by surprise, devastating me. It brought up too many emotions. I felt strongly at that moment that I could never date Kathy without bringing up emotional juxtapositions. Of course, I got over that, but it took a lot of time. In a similar way, I also felt for *Kathie's* family, who eventually were present in force at our wedding, witnessing another wedding with a Kathy and Gary. They took it amazingly well.

Friends

We became friends immediately and stayed very close. At a group pool party, even though we were both dating other people, some of our friends noticed that we seemed to be together in a more than platonic way. But we were very good little girls and boys during those years. We never kissed passionately. So on our first date, we felt like we'd been together for a long time.

Kathy and I had lunch a few times. One day, at Hamburger Hamlet, I told her outright that I could never date her because her three boys were too far out of my experience, understanding and comfort area. I was a daughter person and didn't know what to do with three very active, precocious boys. Very different. I did not want to fail as a boy's dad. So I had to overcome that issue. I sensed a little interest on her part, and I didn't want to mislead her. I felt that Kathy probably liked me at least enough to date me if the situation ever came up, but I did not want to mislead her, so I eliminated the possibility. Remember, I am a relationship person. I wouldn't start with someone knowing that it could not go further than dating.

During this time, Kathy and I had lunch or dinner a few more times, usually with other people and when my current relationship was on the rocks. We would go to dinner and a movie, sometimes with other people. We were both dating other people, even if the relationships might be temporarily on hiatus, so we felt unconditionally committed to the idea of trust and loyalty. This served to strengthen the trust in our own relationship right from the beginning. It was worth the wait.

We saw each other at social functions, support group meetings, and some classes, all perfectly brother/sister. Well, brother/sister in actions, not in thoughts. There was always an unspoken bond between us that went beyond the casual nature of these meetings.

As each of us dated other people, we often talked over the phone. I was fighting at least two things. One was my attraction to her. The other was my utter horror at the way her boys treated her, and her inability to handle the situation. This problem, to one degree or another, may not be uncommon, but it was new to me. The boys had undergone a major trauma, and were deeply scarred. I could hear loud, sustained commotion in the background during every phone conversation, and this regularly turned ugly and verbally abusive toward Kathy. Anything that she wanted them to do was met with an immediate, "No." The verbal abuse was what they had apparently observed from their father, for which no one had ever seen any consequences. Later I saw that in spite of their troubled frame of reference, they also have a sweet nature. Part of my job would eventually be to try to help the boys through the bad and more into the good, and away from the self-defeating, if they would let me in. I wasn't even thinking of the perilous journey with a family of four teenagers at one time, with Ellie having grown into her twenties by then. I guess it's a good thing that I was not that far sighted!

The boys: Did someone say "blended family?"

Kathy was bucking the boys' conditioning and the various factors that molded them during their formative years. The boys really needed a dad who would show them how to respect women, especially their mom, as well as each other and themselves.

The Big Brother program provided three outstanding matches for the boys. Better matches could never have been made. Each of the sensitive, patient, generous men is still significant in their lives. But that wasn't enough. I felt that they needed a big, tall, loud man who was passionately involved with playing sports. I was none of these things. I'm small, quiet, physically strong, fit and active, but not into sports because of eye and back problems, with main interests in the arts and philosophy. My intellectual pursuits conflicted with their prime directive of sports, in which they excel and in which I never did. The actor in me, however, presented a picture of an immaturity that was compatible and complementary with their interests. And it did turn out to work for us a little. I would have a lot of work to do in any case. My sensitivity would be good for the boys, but would they ever identify with a man who was more into intellectual pursuits? They would be taller than I by the time they were fourteen. Taller, yes, but they would have to be older than fourteen to beat me in arm wrestling.

So I was concerned that my interests and abilities might not be compatible with theirs, or looking at it more positively, it might present a real growth opportunity for both them and me.

My girls were quiet, like my whole life up to that point. They were sensitive and caring of my feelings, just the opposite of the boy's reaction to things. They were easy. I really looked forward to seeing my girls, and Kathy, who loves her boys unconditionally, also looked forward to seeing her sons but very frequently dreaded their onslaught.

I joined the boys in some activities, such as soccer games, the *Cirque du Soleil*, movies, air shows, to try to find some common ground. I am still working on that part. We would not be totally compatible, but with time, and as we grew closer during lulls in the war, it would not be hard at all to love them. Dads and sons never get along one hundred percent anyway. I had traits that they had not seen before that would be good for them, even though this would be perceived at first as either weakness or an adversarial position. It would be a significant conflict for me. Did I want so much negativity? I had a choice at that time. I *could* have opted out. But I couldn't opt out. I was in love with Kathy who brought so much into my life that was positive. It far outweighed the conflict, most of the time. And anyway, life is full of conflict, and joining with this family would mean that I would never have a boring life. I see that as more positive than negative. It's the embodiment of the upside of the Chinese curse, "...may you live in interesting times."

If the boys seem like perfect horrors, remember, they are boys. They are damaged from their circumstances, but within a more whole family, they are slowly coming around. They now are beginning to understand about kindness toward their mother, and placing their anger in an appropriately controlled way, at least to minimize physical danger. During their young lives, they were not given behavioral parameters, and Kathy could not control them alone. Kathy did her share of denying the problem from time to time. Discipline was a skill that would take a long time for her to learn. They still have a lot to work out from their loss and the abusive behavior that they apparently witnessed, which was a part of their early education. But at least now they have someone with whom to work these things out. But the question haunted me: could I unconditionally love someone whose behavior was so foreign to me? Yes. Whatever the anthropological explanation might be, throughout all of the posturing, adolescent acting out and assorted nonsense, I do love them. And upon careful intro-spection into my own childhood, much of the behavior that seemed foreign, was actually familiar.

Like most families, the three boys have distinctly different personalities, each with distinct talents, and each will take a sep-arate path in life.

After our marriage, as I began to get back into my profes-sion and comfort zone while exploring common ground with my new family, I performed a children's show at the Armand Ham-mer Museum in Westwood, near UCLA. I was able to incorporate each of my children into the show. We acted together and did daddy/child jokes between routines. It was fun and a nice family experience, with Kathy in the act from the audience. We were all able to be immature together. I discovered what I already knew. I would exploit that immaturity or playfulness in myself, and ex-tend it to the children as much as possible.

Dating Kathy

So, one day Kathy and I found ourselves both unattached at the same time. I was trying very hard not to date her and did a real "job" on myself to convince myself that I would not, could not, should not date her, all the while knowing that I was protest-ing too much and that there was no way to avoid dating her. At first, I felt sure that the boys would be impossible for me and that I might do them harm through my inability to be an effective father to them. But it happened despite my efforts and self-cajoling to the contrary. We had one of our platonic dinners with Gail, one of our widow friends, who had just met the man of her dreams. She left us to our own devices at the end of the evening, something that had never happened before, and the result was the beginning of our relationship.

We stopped for coffee and made chit chat, while my mind was racing. I was thinking, "Don't ask her out. Don't ask her out!" At the same time, I heard myself say, "Well, do you want to give it a try?" So my mouth knew more than I did. The way I talk inappropriately at times, it seems like my mouth can be a real dummy at times. This time it was very wise. Well, she said yes, and, surprise, surprise, I was excited. I had only wanted to do that for three years already. I guess a little excitement is an appropriate reaction.

I took her home and we were standing by her garage. So we said good night, with plans to see each other alone, on a real date, with no commitments to get in our way. The classic question came up at that time. To kiss or not to kiss. This wasn't really a date, after all. It was a pre-date or an evolved practice date. On the other hand, we had known each other as great friends for three years and had never kissed. As the reasoning was going through my mind, my wise mouth knew what to do. We were kissing before I got a chance to finish speculating why it was or wasn't okay. It was a little cautious, not fully committed at first, but it was effective. After all, I had wanted to do that for three years! So that led to the second kiss, and the third, and more. But who's counting? Perhaps Kathy's housekeeper, Marta. During all of this new exploration and smooching, well, more than smooching, Marta was standing there, watching it all, enjoying it, but not knowing what to do or say. All she wanted to do was take out the trash. And she was trapped, but mesmerized. We were sufficiently embarrassed until we remembered that we were actually adults and we were doing nothing wrong, nor were we sneaking around. So Marta did her thing and we all laughed and smiled, and then Kathy and I resumed saying, "Good night," "Very good night," and "Excellent night."

I started our dating cautiously at first, still trying to talk myself out of it, but I knew. I met a few women for coffee or an informal date, to be sure I wasn't on the rebound from Carla. I was also still unsure of my interactions with the boys and trying to work it out in my mind. At the end of that process, I did find one woman to be very interesting, although not on a relationship basis. Kathy was dating other people too, and about the time that I met **Vicky** and started to find her intellectually interesting, Kathy found herself being wooed seriously by a very persistent man. He showered her with gifts right from the start and succeeded in snowing her, indicating his hunger for marriage within the first few days. Kathy was flattered, of course. Regardless of his obvious compulsiveness and questionable sincerity, it upped the ante and I saw Kathy about to make another serious mistake, partly due to my indecision. I weighed the factors, ran the scenarios in my mind and came up with the non-scientific and totally appropriate emotional response, "To hell with everything non-emotional. What do you feel? What if she were out of your life? How long have you been friends and what does that mean? Just shut up and marry her, dummy." I was more than a little aware that I was taking a big risk with my lifestyle, with the complication of raising three boys, for a total of five children, but life is a risk, and some risks being more fun than others.

The proposal

We had dated exclusively for about six months when I began to think about how I would propose to her. Running a few scenarios together, I resolved not to rehearse what I was going to say. It had to be completely of the moment, from the heart. We were at the Inn of the Seventh Ray in Topanga, outside of Los Angeles, which that night was typically romantic. Kathy had no idea that I was going to ask her that night, or ever, for that matter. In fact, I think that she had recently accepted the unlikelihood of ever hearing a proposal from me. We lifted our wine glasses, as we often did before a meal, and made our usual toast. Usually it was "to us." Very simple. Tonight it was a little different. I looked her solidly in the eyes and added a second toast. "To the rest of our lives together." Kathy blinked.

"What did you say?"

"You didn't hear me?"

"I heard you. I just want you to say it again."

"To the rest of our lives together."

"Do you mean it? Now her eyes were glistening, and so were mine.

I felt like saying that she had to answer me before the salad came, so I wouldn't have to pay for it if she said no. I often have these weird thoughts. But I knew the answer, and it came just the way I wanted it.

"What about the boys?" Kathy knew well about the conflict and that this was a package deal.

I gulped and answered in my usual verbose manner. "I'll do my best to make it work. My love for you is stronger than the potential downside. We'll work it out. I don't know how yet, but we will." That's all we can do in life.

The salad was safe.

Deciding to come into the children's' lives was not a decision done haphazardly. It took a year of being with them literally every day before I was able to summon the courage to commit to them. I was going to ask Kathy to marry me on New Year's Eve, but we were derailed by an incident involving one of the boys. Kathy and I embraced him literally and figuratively, and formed a tight, if still fragile bond, turning this into a moment with some upside. Still, this new experience freaked me out a little, and caused me to rethink for three months.

But once I gave into the emotional bond and the loving support that she had already given me, committing to Kathy was easy. That's what did it, actually. Life is not a safe condition. Taking a chance, taking a risk was part of what we do everyday when we get out of bed. A larger risk was worth the upside, which is my relationship with Kathy and my unconditional love for my new family, despite the adjustments.

My traumatized persona, still healing from the life rupture of a few years before, caused me to really think this one through. I was apprehensive about how I would adjust to this condition so different than almost fifty years of my life. Stimulating proposition, no? Yes, and it's working. Not easy! Definitely not perfect, whatever that word means. Each day presents its own challenges requiring patience, creativity, logistics and energy, proving to be quite difficult at times, but not dull!

It's a shock when your dream crashes down and buries you emotionally. I had a hard time reviving my emotional life and dealing with reality versus the ideal. The ideal came in two increments. The first involved removing *Kathie* from the perfect pedestal upon which no one could compete. The second was the search for a new relationship. I tried to keep my relationships on a realistic level, but a little idealism works as well now as it did with my first wife. The life that I have now is as close to ideal as I could ever imagine, even with its very interesting reality reminders!

The children react to the engagement

All of the children reacted to our engagement very enthusiastically. Their body language showed the relief of a great burden. The boys were fairly sure that they had "screwed up" any chance of a marriage by their actions. But I also saw their potential. The girls were always sure I would propose to Kathy and felt that if I hadn't, I would have been a prime idiot. They told me that afterwards.

On the surface it appears that it took longer for the older children to acclimate. This is normal, since they were with their original parent longer. I get a real thrill when the boys call me Dad. It's one of the biggest compliments that anyone could give me, but I never suggested that they call me that. I felt that such a request would be inappropriate, given the circumstances, and it would have been wrong of me to place that emotional pressure on them. They are warm and affectionate in their own ways when they are not being monsters. Well, the *lovely* teenage years present the quest for independence, acting out, and communication shut down. Their personalities are quite explosive. We butt heads a lot, but they are finding behavior parameters. So there's hope that they will be survivors, and not self-destructive. There is a germ of health-consciousness (pardon the pun), and I eagerly await the day that they discover the concept known as The Future. I'm told that they would be butting heads far worse with their natural father, but I studiously avoid comparing or saying anything negative about their natural father, since I only know him through the words of others. I'm learning about genetics vs. environmental influences in child rearing. Despite this chasm, which can only be partly breached, I do have the answer to my question: I do love the boys unconditionally. I get really pissed at them, and they at me, but the love remains. That makes me a moderately strict father, but a real pushover when the boys show that they are willing to work on their problems, accept responsibility for their actions, and listen to those who would try to protect them from a tendency toward self-punishment.

The Wedding

When it came to making the plans for the wedding, I briefly had thoughts about an ideal image versus the probable reality of the day. I had a generalized picture in my mind of a perfect wedding/honeymoon. Those pictures rarely resemble reality once the day arrives. Little things can become over-emphasized under the circumstances, and they can intrude to spoil your fun, if you don't keep your perspective. I needed to put a damper on my idealized expectations, which could have set me up for failure. I decided to take the day moment-to-moment and not let individual problems cast a pall over the day. During that day, upon remembrance, I can't think of a single meaningful negative moment among all of the love and support. I was intensely joyful at this new beginning. It would have been very difficult to spoil that.

The ceremony and honeymoon went far better than my best expectations. I've never had so much fun in my life. Of course, we often talk about it. The deaths and aftermath seemed like a dream from which we could not awaken. Now, in stark contrast, this moment was like a dream, but one from which we don't want to awaken, and in many ways I still live this dream.

Dr. John Sherwood officiated. He would have been a terrier had he been a dog, no offense meant. He was good for us because he is a serious man who could also make us laugh. He understood what we had been through because he had also been a young widower, now happily remarried. I'm uncomfortable with the deadly serious nature of many weddings. It's understandable, but the formality can look like funerals if you are as overly sensitive as I am. And this ceremony contrasts completely with that image. The ceremony went smoothly and comfortably. We were loose and there were lots of smiles and tears in the audience. We knew that there would be an abundance of tears, given that all four families and all of the friends that helped us through our difficulties were there, so having a respectful but completely upbeat ceremony was important.

The crushing of the wine glass at the end of the ceremony, felt like a clean break from the sadness and the need to dwell on the past. This new beginning enhanced the permission and ability to put the past in the proper perspective, part of what made me what I am today. These things had already happened, and a wedding is not needed for everyone in order for this state to be achieved, but this moment felt symbolic of that graduation.

When Dr. Sherwood put the glass on the floor for me to

crush, he said, "Now wait a second so I can get my hand out of the way, and don't bang too hard."

I waited, but I found myself welling up emotionally, as I had been throughout the ceremony, and my foot crashed down on the glass, hard. With a loud crack, the glass, not the hand, broke nicely and both my foot and I were quite happy. Everyone in the room understood my forcefulness.

For me, this moment represented the end of the journey from tragedy to healing and of the part of my life, which I will always cherish as a rich memory, to the beginning of an optimistic future. I felt proud, excited and lucky to be cementing a bond with a woman as positive and caring as Kathy. I felt the bond of new friends whom I met because of Kathy. I felt the love of both of my in-law families and my own mother and step-dad. I could sense the unseen presence and approving nods from our departed loved ones. I felt my growing religious enlightenment, the official end of ten years of sadness, including *Kathie's* illness, and the final statement of permission to go on. And I was having fun!

Kathy and her parents planned most of the wedding. The room was light and cheery and the staff knew what they were doing. The Deejay was just the right blend of experience and improvisation with irreverent wit. The food was probably good, but I don't remember eating it. I wore a morning coat for the first time. I really felt like dressing up. And Kathy, in her white wedding dress, reminded me of Jane Seymour in the movie, *Somewhere in Time*. Her look was radiant, classic, soft, nostalgic, timeless, beautiful, perfect. The main thought in my mind was that I was having the greatest day of my life. The overwhelming feeling in my heart and radiating throughout my body, was love for Kathy and joyfulness in that state. I couldn't get enough of her. I still can't.

We had extraordinary fun and soaked up love and good wishes from friends and families, including both original in-law families. They really are not former in-law families. They're still a very important and immediate part of our lives. How lucky we are for that! Seventeen people from my first wife's family were there, from the mid-west and the east coast. Of course we've been there for them also. I think it is especially impressive because it is so hard to lose a daughter and sister, etc. They fully accepted seeing me with another Kathy, even though it's spelled differently.

The same acceptance is true with Kathy's first in-laws. I am happy to be part of their family. They have been so accepting of me, and so much fun to know.

Kathie's family know me enough to understand that she is not being replaced, but I am moving on, just as she would have admonished me to do.

The honeymoon

The honeymoon started with a one-hour drive to the Simpson House, a beautiful, romantic Bed and Breakfast in Santa Barbara. I reserved a cottage for one night. We soaked in bubbles that night, took in hors d'oeuves and sipped a very interesting wine blend, and got to sleep late. Don't worry, she was gentle with me.

We drove up the coast highway the next day, stopping for lunch at a quaint, Laura Ashley style restaurant/inn called the Apple Farm, one of my family's favorites. We had an outdoor lunch and then continued up the coast, past San Simeon, the Hearst Castle, and up to Big Sur. The Ventana Inn was waiting for us, secluded in the hills. We were above the fog, which looked like a floating, gently rolling sea of steam. The weather was ideal for lolling in the hot tubs at night, sipping champagne and counting the many shooting stars, by the pool during the day, and hiking and exploring Big Sur and nearby Carmel. We enjoyed some romantic dinners, including a meal of Halibut cheeks, a very tender and tasty part of the fish which I had never seen before and haven't since. My mother and stepfather stayed with the children, brave souls.

We sat in our robes on our balcony at the Ventana, sipping champagne with a strawberry inside the glass. We had just returned from a very relaxing hot tub. We had been counting shooting stars in the hot tub and continued on the balcony, happy and absolutely sure that we were where we wanted to be, and that it was right for us. Our bond had been formed starting four years before. The wedding and honeymoon cemented the bond, and through the good and the bad, we are still experiencing growth and closeness, and, yes, we are finishing each other's sentences, and even starting them. And when we argue, we are able to get back to the good stuff. Not idealistic, but reality in the best sense.

About one month later, it was school time and again time to fill out papers. I had a moment of pause. No longer widowed, I checked, "Married." And to a wonderful, sensitive, beautiful, cute, funny, sexy one at that...oops, I have to fill out school papers! It was another happy reminder and a contrast with the sad reminders of the recent past. Happy, married, and yet still aware that it *all* happened, and that I still feel sad for my loss, even within the happy times. That is life, after all. And it is up to me to see the glass as half-full. Fortunately, with Kathy, it's easy.

Who do you love?

Love is a completely mystifying and complicated condition and process. The many kinds of love encompass fraternal, paternal, maternal, courtly, passionate, selfless, and mature. Love between a man and a woman can encompass few, many or all of these categories of love.

People ask me if I loved *Kathie*. I loved her very much. But that is not what the people were really asking me after she had been gone for a few years. Do I love her or am I *in love* with her? Being in love implies immediacy, urgency, whereas mature love can be a fulfillment and reciprocation of a need. At its best, romantic love is an intimate sharing between two partners, both caring about the other's needs and point of view.

Kathie and I were married nineteen years and eleven months. We were together for two years before that. We were truly partners, sharing almost everything.

Before *Kathie* became ill, we had reached the point where we loved each other but were not infatuated. There was a true sharing and a mutual enjoyment of life, issues, events and each other, but there was no immediacy. We knew that we loved each other and that there was no known threat to us, or our marriage.

After she became ill, everything changed for me. My love heated back to the urgent stage, with a poignant reminder of what I had and what I stood to lose.

After she died, that urgency compounded. It took months to process the reality of her passing and fall out of urgent love and back into mature love. The dreams about *Kathie* helped that process, as did time itself, and the hard work processing my grief.

However, the mature love that I now felt was different

than the mature love that I felt when we were married. We were no longer together and could never be, at least on this earth. I could never hold her, kiss her, ask for her counseling, or share a joke. It was a somewhat romanticized memory with an instinctive but intellectually clouded acknowledgement that we were once so close that we will always be close in some way.

I understood that I had enjoyed more love than most people are lucky enough to experience in their lifetime. I should be grateful, and this might have mediated my suffering some, except that I also lost so much.

The hard job of dealing with reality had to be finished before I could move on to other possibilities. *Kathie* was gone. But she was not gone from my memory. She was not absent from the glue that held me together and from my self-definition, the sum of my experiences throughout my life. With a gut-wrenching process, I needed to bring myself to the point where both *Kathie* and I gave me permission to be alive, even though she was not.

Now, how do I feel? It has been more than ten years since *Kathie* died. I don't want *Kathie* to go away completely. That would negate a large portion of the best part of me.

But how do I feel? I have a new life partner. Now, without guilt, I have allowed myself to experience the sharing and the coming together with another person. Things are very different with Kathy, but one familiar thing exists. I am deeply in love with Kathy, experiencing the urgency, the passion, the warmth, the laughter, the mature love. Being with Kathy means being connected with life on the highest plane. If I was lucky once, I am incredibly lucky this time.

I love *Kathie*, but I am in love with Kathy. This might be confusing, even to a person with a split personality! Kathy has my fullest attention and life with her has been good. Perfect? I don't even know what that word means. Of course, there are superficial issues between us. There were issues with *Kathie*, too. But for me, yes, perfect. We are true partners and we are holding on tightly. We know what can happen. And we do not take each other for granted, which is another lesson learned the hard way. Every day is a gift

PART TWO:
KATHY'S STORY

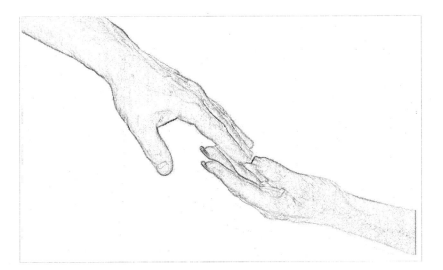

Chapter 8:
THE HAPPY ENDING

I looked up into the magnificent array of stars in the clear night sky above Big Sur on August 1, 1995. Not one, but eight shooting stars in a period of one hour, magically illuminated the sky. It wasn't so urgent to make a wish because, finally, my wishes and dreams had come true. This brilliant occurrence was a "sign" that life would finally be good again, even better than before...

Chapter 9:
THE EARLY YEARS

I was a twenty-three year old elementary school teacher in Los Angeles, when we met in the summer of 1976. I went to Michigan to attend a cousin's wedding and met Sandy through another cousin. Sandy was dashingly handsome and we had immediate chemistry.

He was loving, caring, generous, and very charming. It troubled me that he smoked, because my grandfather had died of a smoking related illness. However, because my life until then had been so blessed with good fortune, it seemed as if nothing bad could ever happen to me or those close to me.

We continued to talk for hours every night, and became engaged that December while I was in Michigan visiting. We planned the wedding for July 3, 1977. Sandy was in Michigan and I was in Los Angeles. Our daily phone conversations and our four brief visits, convinced me that he was the perfect mate for me, even though this was a classic long-distance relationship. My parents and friends felt that it was difficult to really know a person unless you were with them on a continual basis. Of course, I disagreed. My father, a notable physician, also predicted that Sandy would develop some kind of malignancy at an early age if he did not change his unhealthful eating and his habitual smoking.

Marriage
When we were married, we really didn't know each other very well. When we would rendezvous, we were both on our very best behavior, and I thought that this flawless relationship would

never change.

I was shocked to see Sandy's impulsive, volatile temper. At our California wedding he cruelly insulted his aunt, causing extreme distress to the rest of the family. By the time the wedding was over, few relatives from Sandy's side wanted anything to do with him.

Sandy was still angry about the events of the wedding and it put quite a damper on our honeymoon, which consisted of a drive from Los Angeles, back to Michigan, where we were to live. Gazing out of the car window, I became increasingly ill at ease, wondering if this marriage was going to work.

Once we were married, after a discussion about smoking, he snapped at me and said that he would stop smoking when he felt like it, *not* when he was told.

To my great joy, I became pregnant in 1980. It took him a while to adjust to the pregnancy.

Sandy's volatility

Sandy's quick temper never mellowed and his verbal abuse towards me escalated over time. He could be very cruel and say horrible, hurtful things. Soon thereafter, he would forget how cruel he had been and become charming, sweet, and warm. Living with him was an emotional roller coaster. I learned quickly that the way to get along with him was to never fight, argue, or disagree. This was true for friends as well. If a friend said something that Sandy didn't like, he'd stop speaking to them, often after insulting them. Friends who were verbally abused by Sandy, or who saw me verbally abused, often questioned why I would stay in such a relationship.

Commitment to this marriage was very important to me, so even though there were many times when I was not happy or fulfilled, I did love him. I knew the loving and caring side of him as well, so I always hoped that things would get better. I also hung on because I was afraid to be alone and I didn't have the self-respect and confidence to feel that I could be totally independent.

Soon after our marriage, I realized that I did not really know Sandy when I married him. During our long distance courtship, I had not seen his moodiness, his extremely short temper, or his disrespectful attitude. When Sandy was in a good mood, he was the kindest, most lovable man on earth, with a fabulous sense of humor. He was a generous man, overwhelming me with beautiful jewelry and clothing. In fact, he was so generous that he would give a friend or family member his last dollar if they needed it. He told me often how much he adored and loved me, even right after verbally abusing me. As abusive as Sandy could be to those he loved and cared about, his abusiveness never extended to his work. He had a wonderful reputation in his building business and never had a problem getting along with his clients. He was a perfectionist, taking great pride in his work. I was very proud of that.

A strange prediction

So many things just can't be adequately explained. In 1979, two years after Sandy and I were married, his mother passed away. She was a lovely woman and I still miss her. Following the funeral, everyone went back to my sister-in-law's house to pay respects. I met Belva, Sheila's housekeeper, for the first time, having heard about her psychic abilities. As I introduced myself, I could see that Belva was not only looking at me, but all around me. She told me that I had a vibrant aura. Then she shocked me by telling me that Sandy would not be my only husband. She told me that I would have two marriages and that I would have three boys and two girls. This sounded absolutely ludicrous. As much as I loved children, I never thought that I would have five of them. This encounter was rather eerie and unsettling to me and of course I never mentioned it to Sandy or Sheila. I forgot about it until after Gary and I were married, with three boys and two girls. I called Sheila the day after my recollection and she told me that Belva was so successful at predicting the future, that she no longer did housekeeping and was featured on many local Detroit TV shows.

Living in Michigan

While living in Michigan, I was teaching elementary school and teaching guitar in the evenings and weekends to help make money. I worked hard because Sandy's building business was doing poorly and Sandy was at home, not making much money.

Jamie

Our first son, Jamie Erron Smith, was born on July 24, 1981, exactly one month after his scheduled due date. We started to wonder if he was ever going to come out! When he finally did arrive, Sandy was ecstatic. He had taken the Lamaze class with me and helped me through the natural childbirth. The moment Jamie entered this world, Sandy cried like a baby.

Sandy was very loving and attentive while I was in the hospital, but when I came home, even though I was very weak and had some tearing during the birth, he expected me to clean the cat's litter and feed her. My mother confronted Sandy. "How dare you expect Kathy to do that job when she was ordered by the doctor to stay off of her feet." Sandy blew up at her, caused her to cry and told her to leave. He was quite rude to both of my parents. This was supposed to be one of the happiest times of our lives, and he ruined it. Eventually, he did realize how cruel he had been, and he did apologize. He just had a short fuse and never learned to think before he lashed out at people. My parents, realizing that he was basically a good person, always accepted his apologies.

Self-image

Sandy could have profited from a little psychiatric help for anger management. Whenever I suggested this to him, he would snap at me and tell me that he was fine. Everybody else, including me, had a problem, not him. What could I say?

Sandy was concerned about his self-image, and that was far more important to him than the comfort or safety of his family. He still insisted that we drive corvettes even though it was dangerous to transport an infant when three of us were in the car. I felt badly that my husband valued materialistic things more than anything else. I was so much the opposite, having been raised with an appreciation of the arts and travel, with less emphasis placed on materialism.

My travels-why I never take anything for granted

While I was in college, I was very fortunate to have been given the opportunity to travel with my parents throughout Europe, Asia, and the Orient. The highlight of my travels took place over two summers in the early seventies volunteering with Care/Medico in the hospitals of the underdeveloped and underprivileged countries of Afghanistan and Indonesia. My father volunteered to teach the doctors and treat patients there, while my mother organized the pharmacies, and I worked with the pre and post-operative children. I quickly learned from these enriching experiences, to appreciate life to the fullest and to be thankful for the comforts that we take so much for granted here in this country.

The move to California

Sandy's building business continued to do poorly. I suggested that we move to California where the employment opportunities might be better, and I would be able to be with my immediate family again. He agreed, feeling that the change would do us all good, so we moved from Detroit to California in the beginning of 1982.

After three months of living with my parents, we found a lovely two bedroom, two-bathroom apartment in Sherman Oaks. We became the resident managers of that thirty-six-unit apartment. Having built and managed his own apartments in Michigan, Sandy taught me the property management business, which enabled me to become the landlord's property supervisor in charge of five apartment buildings, as well as commercial and industrial buildings. I was able to manage this job without ever having to put my children in daycare.

Adam

In the beginning of January, 1984, I became pregnant with our second child. Sandy sold his Corvette, and bought a very expensive Cadillac, with high car payments. I was furious. I wanted a more practical car, so we could begin to save some money. This was the only way that we could ever save enough money to buy our own home. That wasn't important to Sandy. The car was.

Our second son, Adam Brandon Smith, was born on September 18, 1984, three days before his due date. We were elated. Sandy, who cried for joy when Jamie was born, laughed for joy this time.

The unhealthy lifestyle

Sandy continued to smoke heavily and eat unhealthfully. He said that he enjoyed smoking. "So what if I die in my sixties. You'll have the insurance." He was not concerned about the hazards of the secondary smoke. There just was no reasoning with him.

It seemed that we never did the things that made me happy, such as saving for a better home for the family rather than owning two Corvettes and a Cadillac. It was always what Sandy wanted, despite my objections and valid criticism. I always gave in because it was futile to fight, and intimidating. In order to keep this marriage together, I was the one who was going to have to bend. Sometimes I think that maybe it was better that he had his way since his life was so short.

Sandy finally consented to smoking only outdoors or in the privacy of our bathroom. I pointed out to him that smoking in an enclosed, damp space with no ventilation, was very dangerous. It was repulsive to me as I watched the walls and ceilings of the bathroom become discolored to a dull brown with dark spots. The cigarette odor permeated the room as well. I felt helpless. It was a losing battle, so I tried to concentrate on our children and myself.

Finally, it seemed that our luck might begin to change. Sandy was contracted to build a 16,000 sq. ft. home in Bel Air.

We moved into a rental townhouse in a community which frowned upon children. If only Sandy had thought more of his family rather than his own gratification over tennis courts and a large community pool. Then to further kill our plans for moving into our own home, he traded in the Cadillac and bought a Mercedes. Sandy purchased it with payments of almost $700 a month. Then a few months before the birth of our third child, Sandy decided to purchase a run down apartment building in Hollywood. It was more than fifty years old, and in a terrible area. But he told me that he knew what was best and he felt that it would throw off some good income. That decision would return to haunt me.

Jordan

Our third son, Jordan Alexander Smith, arrived on his due

date, April 14, 1987. Sandy was very attentive and excited.

Sandy laughed and cried this time. He was truly thrilled with his three sons. He thanked me for giving him these beautiful, precious children and he told me how much he loved me. He turned out to be a wonderful and attentive father, always involved in their extra-curricular activities.

My parents were thrilled for us, and continued to be very loving and attentive grandparents. I was grateful to have them nearby.

Sandy's Work

Through his developing West Coast reputation, Sandy was contracted to build his second mansion in Bel Air. This time, 12,000 sq. ft. He finally started to talk about perhaps buying our own home. I was delighted that he was finally coming to his senses about providing a more suitable living space for his family of five. Sandy always talked about building a home for us but he was adamant that the site be a prime location with an excellent view. He would not hear of moving into a more modest home until we could afford better. Since we couldn't afford his ideal site, he was content living in the rented townhouse, despite the difficulties that we faced living there with children. Had he not bought Corvettes, a Cadillac, a Mercedes, and a more than fifty-year-old apartment building, we would have lived so much more comfortably. His professional abilities and talents certainly didn't extend to his personal financial decisions.

Don't rock the boat

Looking back now, I really wasn't very forceful. But in order to save the marriage, I felt I couldn't be strong. Knowing how unhappy and dissatisfied he made me at times, Sandy warned me that if I ever left him he would make my life miserable. He told me that after having three children, I would be considered "used goods" and no man would want me. These threats terrified me, and the degrading comments slowly but surely, tore down my confidence. I was more convinced than ever that I could not survive on my own if I had chosen to leave him.

When Sandy finally looked at homes for us, he only viewed homes that were priced so above our means that we could never realistically make the payments, let alone have enough for a down payment. He just wasn't rational. When I would attempt to bring him back to reason, he would simply say to the children, "Your mother doesn't want us to have a nice home. It's her fault that we are still in apartments."

These comments were not fair and so untrue. Comments of this sort planted the seeds of resentment against me in our children, and the way that Sandy spoke to me in front of the children set the stage for their disrespectful attitude toward me. Dealing with their disrespectful attitude is still an issue that has not been fully resolved.

The boat begins to founder

Around the end of 1990, Sandy seemed to be coughing more and developed terrible headaches from the severe coughing attacks. I pressured him to go to his internist for a check up. He wouldn't listen to me. He knew something was very wrong and he was frightened by the thought of what the doctor might find.

Chapter 10: ILLNESS

The cough

After two months, Sandy's coughing was much worse and he was having great difficulty breathing. Finally, in January, 1991, he went to see his internist. The chest X-ray showed something on the lung. Sandy called me from the doctor's office and told me that he would be home late because he was being sent to a pulmonary specialist to have a CT Scan of his lungs. Things were happening alarmingly fast, but ironically, the time seemed to pass in slow motion.

Finally, Sandy arrived home at around 7:30 P.M., terribly distressed. The CT Scan showed something blocking part of his right bronchial tube. The next morning he was to be admitted to Cedars Sinai Hospital for an outpatient procedure called a bronchoscopy.

We couldn't sleep that night. Sandy was very frightened and he couldn't breathe well. I was terrified also, but maintained an outwardly calm manner so I could be reassuring for him. He was now in the doctor's hands and we would do whatever needed to be done to make him well again. I told him that I loved him and was there for him.

Tests and diagnosis

Sandy, our precious three-year-old Jordan, and I arrived at the hospital for the 10:30 A.M. procedure. This involved mild sedation while a tube was inserted down Sandy's throat into the pulmonary cavity. The growth could then be viewed and a biopsy would be taken to determine the nature of the growth.

I anxiously awaited the outcome of the procedure.

At 11:15 A.M. the pulmonary specialist, Dr. Wade, came out of the procedure room and called my name. My heart was beating so hard, I could hear it in my ears, but I'll never forget the doctor's words. "It doesn't look good."

I asked, "Is it a tumor?"

"Yes," he answered.

"And?" I was almost afraid to ask.

The doctor said, " It looks malignant, but we won't know for sure until the biopsy results come back. This will take at least twenty-four hours."

I felt so sad. I looked up at Dr. Wade and said, "I pleaded with him to stop smoking!"

Dr. Wade's response was cryptic. "It's payback time."

My head was spinning and I had a horrible feeling in the pit of my stomach. Crushing feelings of sadness and anger welled up inside me. I recalled Sandy's response to my pleading with him to stop smoking. "Don't ever say 'I told you so.'" I wanted to say it, but I never did.

I followed Dr. Wade, to see Sandy and tell him the news. Sandy was alert, but uncomfortable, and having great difficulty breathing. Sandy said, "Well?"

When Dr. Wade told him, Sandy responded, "Oh shit!" And then he became quiet and just looked out of the window.

He was practically in tears on the way to the car. Dr. Wade scheduled Sandy to be hospitalized at 3:00 P.M. the next day, to try to open his airways.

While we were preparing to leave the hospital following the bronchoscopy, I realized that I had forgotten to have my parking validated. I left Sandy in the car with Jordan while I hurried back to the surgical center. While riding down the elevator on the way back to the car, I broke down and started to cry. A lovely older couple was in the elevator with me. The lovely woman with a sweet smile gently put her hand on my shoulder and said, "You're in pain. God is there with you and you'll be okay."

This statement from a stranger really struck hard. I was in pain and this wasn't a bad dream. It was really happening.

We arrived home from the hospital, and while Sandy was

resting, I made plans with my parents to take care of the children while Sandy and I went to the hospital the next day. My father explained to me that his experience told him the situation didn't look good for Sandy, but there were different treatments that could be tried.

We had a terribly emotional night. We were still hoping that the biopsy would be benign. Sandy knew what was most likely in store for him. That night, I positioned Sandy upright on the living room couch. He was able to breathe more easily this way. I remained on the couch with him, and what an evening it was. Sandy and I both cried. Sandy became almost hysterical. He was so scared. He told me how much he loved us, and the thought of dying and leaving us was just too much to bear. I cried and told him that we wouldn't let him die. He had too much left to do in this world. If he had cancer, then we would deal with it and he would do whatever he had to do to get better. I demanded that he adopt this attitude, and it was the first time in our marriage that he actually listened to me, promising to try to be strong and to get better. As he held me and stroked my hair, he told me that if he didn't make it, he would want me to marry again and be happy. Also, the boys deserved to have a dad. As difficult as it was for him to think of me with another man, he still wanted me to have a life if he could no longer be here.

I was deeply touched and saddened by this conversation. He knew that he really messed up and that he was letting us all down. How pathetic this all was.

Sheila, Sandy's sister, and her husband Alvyn, and our nephew, Randy came over and brought us lunch the next day. Sheila, who worked for Sandy's primary physician, Dr. Lassen, was the person who actually arranged Sandy's upcoming hospitalization. She told us that if the biopsy was malignant, then a very well respected oncologist, Dr. Barry Green, would be called in on the case. We still had no answer on the biopsy, and it was time to leave for the hospital.

Sheila, Alvyn, and Randy accompanied us to the hospital that afternoon. Sandy was admitted and taken to a room and we just sat and waited for the doctor to arrive. Around 4:30, a practical nurse came into the room and told us that Dr. Green would be in shortly. She was shocked when she saw the reaction to her statement. Without knowing it, she had confirmed that Sandy had cancer, because the oncologist was on his way. All of us burst into tears. How could this be happening? Sheila cried, "Oh, my baby brother, oh my baby brother!"

Randy looked bewildered. I was absolutely numb.

I held my poor husband tightly, telling him that I loved him and repeated that we would do what we would have to do.

Around 5:30 P.M. all three of Sandy's doctors, Dr. Lassen, Dr. Wade, and now Dr. Green, came into the room. Dr. Green was a kind, gentle man around the same age as Sandy. He told all of us, that the biopsy showed a small cell carcinoma of the lung. Lung cancer. The bad news was that the cancerous tumor was inoperable. The good news was that this kind of cancer usually responded very well to chemotherapy and radiation. He felt that since Sandy was forty-four years old, he was young enough and strong enough to fight this.

Chemo, more tests and a changed life

Dr. Green told us that he wanted to start Sandy on chemotherapy that evening, and then he would have two more treatments. If he responded, he could go home after the three treatments, and receive the remainder at Dr. Green's office every three weeks, as an outpatient.

Sandy asked, "Dr. Green, could this cancer have been caused by the pollution in Los Angeles?"

"No," Dr. Green answered. "It was directly caused by your cigarette smoking."

The suspense of not knowing was now over, and the doctors painted an optimistic picture for Sandy. He also would be scheduled for a bone scan, and other diagnostic tests, to make sure that the cancer hadn't spread.

We all cried some more. Sandy turned to me, and for the first time ever, apologized for the way he had treated me in the past. Now that he was in a critical health situation, it made him realize how difficult and unappreciative he had been. He promised to change his ways and become a new person. He said that God gave him this second chance, and he was committed to becoming a better, kinder person. Sandy tolerated the first treatment well, which made him somewhat less apprehensive about the next treatment later that day.

Sandy loved his work. He made business calls from the hospital and kept things going despite his absence.

The bone scan and blood work showed that the cancer appeared to be self-contained.

Sandy was still tolerating the chemotherapy and by the time he had the third treatment, there was a real improvement in his breathing. X-rays showed that the tumor was shrinking, which gave us hope for a successful recovery. Sandy told my parents and friends that he was going to be a kinder person. Everyone was happy to hear him sound so good and say such positive things. They knew how difficult Sandy could be, so they were happy to hear that he had finally come to his senses. Friends and family were looking forward to being with the "new" Sandy.

The boys came to the hospital with my parents. They made their dad beautiful Get Well pictures and Sandy cried when he saw them. Oh, how he loved his boys.

Having been told of their dad's illness, the boys were very relieved to see him looking so good and in such a good mood.

The next day Sandy completed the first round of chemotherapy and was released to go home. He had been hospitalized for four days. All of his doctors were very pleased with his improved breathing after the first block treatment of chemotherapy.

The boys were thrilled to see their dad home again. Sandy even went with me to Jamie's soccer practice that afternoon, and went back to work the following day.

We resumed life as usual, and before long, Sandy slipped back into his old abusive ways.

Sandy felt well for the next two weeks, but beginning the third week, he started having difficulty breathing again. At the end of the third week we went to Dr. Green's office for his second course of chemotherapy. We were a little depressed because Sandy seemed to be relapsing. The doctor told us that it was too early to judge the success of the treatment, and that Sandy should never give up. After the course of chemotherapy, radiation therapy would be required as well.

Sandy had the second chemo treatment intravenously in the doctor's office. After the treatment, we returned home and Sandy didn't feel quite as well as he had after the initial treatment. He felt very weak, developed a high fever, and was slightly nauseous. Luckily, the symptoms began to diminish by the next day, although he felt physically drained for a few days.

Sandy continued to work despite his physical condition. I was always impressed with his professional dedication even when he was so ill. By the end of the week following the second treatment, he could breathe more easily and his spirits were lifted again. But like before, by the beginning of the third week, he had trouble breathing again, making him very frustrated and irritable.

The worst emotional scar

Something very traumatic happened one day that would leave our oldest son, Jamie, with emotional scars for many years. One late afternoon, Sandy had come home from the job early because he wasn't feeling well. As he was resting on the living room couch, Sandy abruptly called nine year old Jamie over to him and blurted out, "Jamie, I have cancer and I'm going to die! You will have to take over for me."

Little Jamie just stood there looking at his father silently with tears streaming down his face. Jamie, who always had a terrific sense of humor and an enthusiastic spirit, became very quiet and subdued. This moment changed everything.

Complications

If life with Sandy was difficult before, it was much worse now. His illness and his fear caused him to constantly lash out at me.

The same chemo scenario happened a third time. Sandy would feel good and start to breathe easier after the first week of treatment, and then going into the third week, he would relapse and have difficulty breathing again. X-rays showed that the tumor was shrinking, but not as successfully as Dr. Green had hoped. By the end of the third treatment period, Dr. Green wanted to begin radiation on the tumor. The doctor felt that Sandy's response would be improved by zapping the tumor directly, while maintaining the chemotherapy treatments.

After the first week, the radiation began to totally exhaust him. He was also starting to have difficulty swallowing because his esophagus was within the radiation range. I prepared soft foods for him.

By the third week of radiation, Sandy developed severe burns on his chest and back. I stayed up with him at night putting a variety of creams and lotions on his skin. My poor husband was so uncomfortable. Yet, he never gave up. He even went for his fourth chemo treatment while he was still receiving radiation therapy. That was really hard on him. Again, he continued to work during this painful and debilitating period. When X-rays were retaken it was confirmed that the tumor was shrinking a great deal. That gave us all a big boost and it gave Sandy a renewed positive attitude, motivating him to do what he had to do to get well.

Towards the end of Sandy's radiation treatment, Dr. Green recommended another CT Scan to see if the tumor was gone. To our great relief, the CT Scan showed that the tumor was no longer visible. We were so thrilled.

Sandy wouldn't come to terms with the reality of his situation, so he never made an effort to protect his family by putting his affairs in order if things didn't turn out well. He was responsible for three young boys and a wife who really depended on him. Unfortunately, he cared more about spending money than saving money. Whenever I would suggest that we have a will prepared, he would answer me by saying, "You're already digging my grave." So I dropped the subject.

Throughout Sandy's illness, I was okay as long as I didn't show my fears of the future openly. As I walked our dog alone late at night, I would think about the future and I felt as if I was treading water, panicking, and drowning. I had the ability to snap myself back into the present where my head was once again bobbing above water. This was the only way that I could stay afloat and deal with the inevitable tragedy. I had to take one day at a time. Also, it was my duty to display a strong and cheerful attitude to keep Sandy's spirits up and to keep the children as stress-free as possible, and to maintain a normal life.

Four weeks later, circumstances changed. Sandy was again having great difficulty breathing. When we went to see Dr. Wade, it was confirmed through another bronchoscopy procedure, that Sandy was suffering from Radiation Pneumonitis, a severe inflammation of the lungs caused by the radiation. Sandy was irate and ready to sue all the doctors involved, because he was told that he might never get any better.

Sandy's condition worsened. He was having such difficulty breathing, he was beginning to look cyanotic. I had oxygen delivered to the house, even though he didn't want to deal with it. Soon thereafter he couldn't breathe at all without the oxygen. We had one large tank downstairs by the couch, and when it was time for Sandy to go upstairs to bed, we would drag the extended oxygen tubes up the stairs and into the bedroom. I was always terrified that one of the children would trip over the tubes, cutting off Sandy's oxygen supply.

After a couple days on the oxygen, Sandy seemed to be getting worse. The Friday before Father's Day, I drove him and the oxygen tank to the hospital to be admitted. He was put on a large dose of Prednosone, a steroid that helps inflammation. To the doctors' surprise, Sandy responded so favorably that by Monday he could once again breathe on his own.

While he was in the hospital, blood tests were done, including a radioactive test, which could detect cancer in other parts of the body. By Wednesday of that week, the blood work and other diagnostic tests showed negative results for cancer, so we believed that Sandy was in total remission. He was discharged from the hospital that mid-June day, without oxygen tanks. June went into July and Sandy was doing so well with his breathing that Dr. Wade felt that it was time to gradually lower the dose of the steroid until he was completely off of it.

So, week-by-week we lowered the dose by five mg. Sandy was still breathing well, but he began to experience severe pains in his joints, stomach, and chest. The doctors believed that these pains were caused from the steroid withdrawal.

During the month of July, Sandy was advised to resume a few weeks of oral chemotherapy. He seemed to tolerate the medication just fine, although he still needed pain medication.

In the beginning of August, Sandy went to Dr. Green for some blood work and a short check up. Sandy was still in pain, but his blood work came out normal, and Dr. Green still believed that Sandy's pain was coming from the Prednosone withdrawal.

Now that Sandy could breathe better, he wanted to take the boys and me on a short vacation before school started. He decided to go to Las Vegas between August 13th and 17th. Once we arrived, I knew that Sandy wasn't himself, because he didn't gamble at all. We spent the days relaxing by the pool, enjoying the children, and talking about how we looked forward to future milestones.

Sandy's pain began to get worse and he wasn't able to sleep at night. I would wake up and find him sitting on the edge of the bed, bent over, rocking back and forth. One night, six year old Adam also awakened, and without saying a word, he sat next to his father on the edge of the bed, rocking along side of him. This was a special moment of great compassion and love between father and son. Adam is a very sensitive and loving child and he feels compassion for others.

On the way home from Las Vegas, we stopped for dinner, Sandy ordered a large meal, and couldn't touch it.

Chapter 11: DYING

By the time we arrived home, Sandy was in agony. We called Dr. Green and he told us to continue the present dosage of Prednosone, and he increased the pain medication.

Impaired vision

A few days later, Sandy volunteered to take Adam to a party in Santa Monica so I could take Jordan to another party. I was leery of this idea because I wasn't sure how safe it was for Sandy to be driving. He insisted, so I let him drive. Sandy didn't tell me that he was also experiencing impaired peripheral vision. While he was changing lanes to get on to the freeway, he didn't see a truck in the next lane. The truck side-swiped Sandy and didn't even stop, even though it was Sandy's fault. He arrived safely and Adam made it to his party, but the Corvette was so badly damaged from the accident that it wouldn't start again. While walking to a pay phone to call me, Sandy walked into a telephone pole and scratched his hand badly. When he called me, I felt so horrible that I had given in to his driving. Thank God they were both safe. I then drove to Santa Monica to pick up Sandy and Adam.

We followed the tow truck to Van Nuys, and when we left the Corvette, Sandy never even took a second look at it. This was very alarming since his Corvette was one of his passions. This was another reminder of just how sick Sandy was.

The condition worsens

That Monday, August 19th, I drove Sandy to Dr. Green's

office. I was tormented seeing Sandy in such agony. He could hardly walk at this point.

While at the doctor's office, he began to vomit. Dr. Green decided to take some more blood tests. He told us that perhaps the chemotherapy had caused some chemical imbalance that might be causing the pain. After the blood work was completed, the doctor gave Sandy a shot of Demerol, and I took him home.

Sandy had a night of excruciating pain. Dr. Green called the next morning and told me that Sandy's blood work had shown that his liver function was "way off" and he wanted Sandy to have an ultrasound of his liver, as well as a CT Scan of his brain because of his impaired vision.

Sandy was scheduled for the tests the next day. He had another horrible night and by morning, he could hardly move. I called Dr. Green and told him that it was getting increasingly difficult to manage Sandy at home when he was in so much pain. I was dying inside, watching my poor husband suffer so terribly. It was agreed that if we could wait until Thursday, Sandy could be admitted to the hospital for the tests and pain management.

That Wednesday was pure hell. Sandy was vomiting bile, wasn't eating, and had terrible pain in his stomach and chest. The next morning I helped him into the car. He continually vomited into a garbage bag as I drove to the children's schools to pick them up. While Sandy waited in the car, I ran into the elementary school office. The principal, in a pleasant mood said, "Oh school's just begun and the children are sick already!"

Distraught and depressed, I just blurted out, "No, their father is dying and I have to take them to the hospital with me!" The principal's mouth dropped open. I collected the children and left.

To have actually verbalized what I truly felt about the situation was so frightening to me. Panic began again, but I shut off the outward signs and kept my head above the water by reminding myself to deal with the present time, and not project into the future.

The final days

Finally we arrived at the hospital. Sandy was wheeled up to the cancer ward while I very calmly admitted him. On the way to Sandy's room, as we stepped off of the elevator and turned into the right hallway, the boys and I could hear patients moaning and could see their relatives silently crying.

This was a shocking dose of reality for all of us. Sandy was only forty-four years old, critically ill, and probably dying. This wasn't supposed to happen to a young person with three young children.

The nurses had begun administering a morphine drip to control Sandy's pain.   Later that afternoon, Sandy was awakened for the ultrasound of his liver. The boys and I wheeled him down for the test, and waited there to bring him back up to his room. When Sandy completed the ultrasound, he was in terrible pain again. He was given more morphine and went to sleep. Once Sandy was sleeping and seemed to be more comfortable, I took the children home.

Trying to be calm and maintain normalcy at home, I made a nice dinner, spent time with the children, and put them to bed. Then I called the hospital. The nurse said that Sandy was comfortable and asleep. It was easier for me to sleep knowing that he wasn't suffering at the time.

The next morning was Friday. The telephone rang just as I was leaving to take the children to school. I started shaking, anticipating the doctor's call. It was Dr. Green calling from Sandy's hospital room.   The ultrasound showed that the cancer had spread throughout the liver and, not surprisingly, things didn't look good. However, neither he nor Sandy were ready to throw in the towel yet. The doctor decided to try a very aggressive chemotherapy that wouldn't cure Sandy, but could buy him a little more time.

I was crying and told the doctor not to let Sandy give up hope. I again encouraged Sandy to do what he could to fight this, reminding him of all the reasons to live.

I collected the children and took them to school. While in the car I explained to them that their daddy's cancer was now in his liver and he was going to be on a new chemotherapy. The children were very quiet, each of them deep in thought, and not ready to verbalize what they were feeling. I dropped them off at school and then went directly to the hospital.

I arrived at 9:00 A.M. Sandy was sleeping restlessly. After a while, a nurse came in and started to hook up the new chemotherapy. It was pretty frightening to think how strong the chemo was. The nurse put on a special suit with thick gloves, to protect herself from the toxins.

Sandy was not even aware when the chemo began. He still had not eaten anything, so he was on an IV drip for his nourishment as well as the morphine drip for pain. I just sat at his bedside reading, or doing my property management paper work as he slept. His meals would come and go as he slept.

I had to leave to pick up the children at 3:00 P.M.

My friends were wonderful at this very difficult time. They all lovingly offered their help and support whenever it was needed. They watched the children for extended hours while I was at the hospital, as did my wonderful housekeeper, Marta. My parents, who were out of town at the time, flew back home when they were told of Sandy's deteriorating condition.

The next morning was Saturday. After I returned from coaching Adam's soccer team in Sandy's place, I called the hospital and Sandy's line was busy. I called the nurses' station and was told that Sandy had been very depressed all morning and had taken the phone off the hook himself. The nurse said that he actually sat up in a chair for a while. I hadn't seen him awake since Dr. Green's call Friday morning.

I felt so horrible. Here my husband was sitting up in a chair, probably coming to terms with his fate, and he was alone. My emotional stability was really wavering.

I arrived at the hospital only to find Sandy sleeping again. I saw a blanket and a pillow on the chair. My heart was breaking as I placed the phone receiver back on the cradle. I should have been there. I felt very hurt that he couldn't talk to me and share his fears. We were never able to really speak again.

Sandy slept the rest of Saturday. He became progressively more jaundiced. It frightened me to see him deteriorate so quickly. It was clear that the chemotherapy was not working. Sandy's breathing was becoming more labored. I stayed with him for the rest of the day until late that night, then I went to the market and arrived home around midnight.

Sunday was much the same as Saturday. Sandy slept and I sat by his bedside as his condition continued to worsen. When I arrived home that Sunday evening, I spoke to my dear friends, Marv and Candy. Marv told me that he had gone to the hospital for a few hours and Sandy was awake. He told me that Sandy asked him if he thought he was going to make it. Marv, typically honest and straightforward, told Sandy that he did not believe that he would live. Sandy's response to Marv was that he believed that he had really screwed up his life. He shared his concern about the boys and how they would be after he was gone. I asked Marv if Sandy had said anything about me. He said no.

This encounter made me feel even worse. I should have been the one to have this talk with Sandy. Marv should not have told him that he wasn't going to live. I would have told Sandy that yes, he was very critically ill, and it was likely that he would die, but he was still alive and very much loved and needed. I would have encouraged him not to give up hope.

More depressed than ever, I also felt terribly hurt because Sandy expressed his concern about the boys after his death, yet he had nothing to say about me, his wife. I knew it was selfish for me to feel this way in view of the circumstances, but my emotions were raw. Even though I had tremendous support from my family and friends, I still felt totally isolated. No one could really know what I was going through. I was a thirty-eight-year-old mother with three young children, with a dying husband, in debt and living in a rented townhouse. Soon I would be alone with the tremendous responsibility of being the only parent and provider.

After I tucked the boys into bed, I took Peetie, our dog, for his late-night walk. This was the only time I let myself really feel and actually cry, knowing deep in my heart what was about to happen.

I had problems sleeping that night. I called the hospital nursing station several times during the night, and was told that Sandy was sleeping, but very agitated.

The next morning, Monday, August 26, 1991, I drove the children to school and explained to them that Daddy was still very sick and didn't seem to be getting better. Not one of them said a word. When we got to school they seemed relieved to get out of the car and on to their own lives where they wouldn't have to think about the reality of their father's condition. My parents would pick them up from school and keep them indefinitely.

I arrived at the hospital about 10:30 A.M. As I stepped off the elevator and turned down the hall towards Sandy's room, Dr. Green and Dr. Wade were running ahead of me into Sandy's room. I ran to the room, and what I saw broke my heart. Sandy was attempting to sit up in bed and he was in absolute agony, holding on to his upper right side and stomach area. When he saw me, he uttered the very last words I would ever hear him say to me, "Oh Kath, I'm really bad. I'm really, really bad."

I couldn't speak.

Dr. Green then told Sandy that the pain might be caused from the chemotherapy breaking up all of the cancer tumors. Sandy, looking sad but hopeful said, "Oh, oh, okay, okay."

I started to panic and demanded something stronger for his pain. When he was somewhat more comfortable and sleeping again, I walked the doctors to the elevator. Dr. Wade looked as if he was about to cry. He just looked at me and said, "I'm so sorry. I've never seen anything this bad before. I'm so sorry." Then he quickly stepped into the elevator and I knew that he was having a great deal of difficulty maintaining his composure.

Dr. Green couldn't offer much encouragement. All he could do was apologize and assure me that Sandy would be kept as comfortable as possible.

I felt so helpless. There was just no more hope.

Sandy's lung function was growing increasingly worse, and now his kidneys were no longer functioning. His catheter was filled with solid waste. The urologist was paged. When he arrived and looked at Sandy's catheter, he said out loud, "Why are they wasting my time? There is absolutely nothing that I can do here. He's too far gone." He seemed to be unaware that I was in the room.

When the urologist left, a team of four nurses abruptly entered the room. To my surprise, they passed by Sandy and came to me. They were from Hospice. All I could think as they escorted me to a room down the hall was, "Oh my God, it's a reality. Sandy's dying and there's no more hope."

How was I going to get through this?

I cried out to the nurses, who were very comforting and nurturing, "He couldn't die! How could this happen? Why did he have to smoke? How will I be able to go on living without my husband? My children won't have a father."

All of my pent up emotion began pouring out. One of Sandy's afternoon nurses, Linda, heard me and I was told later that she also broke down and had to spend fifteen minutes in the bathroom pulling herself back together.

When I returned to Sandy's room, Sheila, Alvyn, Randy, and my niece, Pam, were there. I updated them on Sandy's worsening condition and we all cried together. Sheila kept saying, "Come on Little Brother, you gotta hang in. You're my baby brother. You can't die!" As the relatives left, I assured them that I would keep in contact with them.

I called my parents and asked them to keep the children so I could stay. I didn't want Sandy to die alone. My parents wanted to be with me but I felt it was more important for them to be with my children.

Sandy never regained consciousness. I instructed the nurses to keep him appropriately drugged so he wouldn't feel the pain or know what was really going on. Once again, I wanted to bear the pain for him.

As time passed, Sandy's lung function continued to decrease and he was getting more and more agitated as he was unconsciously fighting for air. He was literally drowning in his own fluids. The doctors then gave him a tranquilizer to reduce his agitation. I chose not to have him put on a respirator, since the doctor said that it would only prolong the inevitable.

I felt as if this was all a bad dream or a movie about someone else's tragic life.

My brother, Rick, arrived at the hospital about 9:30 P.M. I was sitting in a chair next to Sandy. When Rick entered the room, he wasn't prepared for what he saw. He freaked out. I had to calm him down and tell him that there was nothing more anybody could do at this point, except to make Sandy as comfortable as possible.

Finally, at 11:00 P.M. Rick leaned over and held Sandy for a minute, told him that he loved him and to "hang in there," and I sent him home.

I continued to sit in the dimly lit room in a chair next to Sandy. The nurses gave me a blanket and a pillow, but I couldn't sleep. Sandy's breathing was so labored. I couldn't believe that he had enough strength left in him to put forth the effort needed to breathe. Every half hour the nurses came in to check his oxygen level, which was decreasing rapidly. The nurse gave Sandy more morphine, to make him more comfortable, and told me that it wouldn't be much longer. It was after 1:00 A.M. and I just couldn't bear his labored breathing any longer. I started to cry. I put my arms around Sandy and told him that it was okay to relax and let go. I told him that he was a real fighter and that he gave it his best, but now it was time to rest. I told him that I loved him.

About 2:00 A.M. I noticed that Sandy's breathing began to change. It was no longer steady. Instead, he would take a deep breath and hold it for ten or fifteen seconds, and then exhale. After about ten minutes of this, as I held his hand, he quietly took a little breath in. And that was it. He was gone.

I gently took the oxygen mask off of his face. It was strange. He no longer seemed to be in his body. He looked like a shell to me. In fact, after I removed the oxygen mask from his face, I looked up at the ceiling and spoke to him. "Sandy," I said as I looked upward, "rest peacefully and never forget how much you were and are loved. We will miss you terribly. Be at peace. I love you."

I then pressed the nurses' button as I stood over my dead husband. After waiting for fifteen minutes, I walked out to the nurses' station. I saw a nurse walking down the hall, and I said, "My husband died fifteen minutes ago."

The nurse said, "Oh my God," and she ran into Sandy's room. He was pronounced dead at 2:30 A.M., August 27th, although I knew that he had died earlier.

I asked the nurse to take the contact lenses out of his eyes. I didn't want him buried in them. I also wanted the lavender silk robe that he was wearing. It was his favorite, and I still have it today.

The nurse then escorted me into a room where I could make calls and she told me that the evening hospital administrator would be in to see me soon, to finish business.

Chapter 12: AFTER

I called my parents first. They asked if I was okay. Functioning on automatic pilot, in a dream-like state, I asked my father what I was supposed to do now. He told me to decide on a mortuary and call them immediately. They took the children to school but did not tell them. That would be my job, once they were home from school.

The immediate necessities

The mortuary representative said that they would pick up "the body." They told me to call after 8:00 A.M. to schedule an appointment to buy a plot, a casket, and plan the funeral.

Then I called Sheila and told her that her brother died. We cried together for what seemed like hours. I told her that I would update her on the funeral plans.

Then I called my brother, Rick, so that he could join me and my parents, to make the plans at the mortuary.

Finally, the hospital administrator came to finalize everything. She couldn't believe that I was alone. She asked if I would be able to drive home in the middle of the night by myself after losing my husband. Feeling totally numb, I told her that I would be okay.

Going home

At around 3:00 A.M. I once again said goodbye to my husband, packed up his things, including his robe and contact lenses, and went down to the parking garage for my car. When I pulled up to the exit gate, the parking attendant demanded more money than what was truly due. I started to argue with him and finally told him that my husband just died, and to please stop hassling me. His response was, "Sure your husband died. What a great excuse!"

I was so angry. I told him it was not an excuse, but a reality. Why else would I be at a hospital at 3:30 in the morning? I paid the ticket, but it was eventually reimbursed to me.

As I drove home down Doheny, to Wilshire, and on to the 405 freeway, I didn't feel as if I was really alone. I felt Sandy's presence very strongly, and I even spoke to him, telling him how much he was loved and how greatly he would be missed.

I arrived home about 4:00 A.M. I showered, washed and dried my hair, and went to bed. The next morning, at around 7:00, after having not really slept, I began to call my friends. They were all very sad and a little shocked. Sandy was the first of our contemporaries to die.

Funeral arrangements

My appointment at the mortuary was at 1:00 P.M. Rick picked me up and then we picked up my parents.

The funeral was scheduled for the next day, Thursday, August 29th, at 1:30 P.M. Jim Kaufman, who married us fourteen years earlier, would bury Sandy.

I then had the horrible task of choosing a coffin. I ended up choosing a solid wood one. I worried about the padding inside. Would it be comfortable? Would it be large enough? These were ridiculous thoughts, but that's what I was thinking.

I felt a little silly asking if there was a dress code. I chose one of his favorite jogging suits, black and white nylon. He had never worn it with a shirt underneath, but I included a white shirt, because I was worried that he would be chilled.

I then had to choose a plot. I remember Sandy telling me in jest, years ago, that if he died first, to make sure that he had a nice view. I chose a beautiful spot near a tree that wasn't too crowded. The view was of rolling hills and even some new construction. He'd feel quite comfortable. I felt very satisfied with my choice.

After finishing up all the details at the mortuary, including the large burial payment, we all got in the car and stopped for lunch. I knew that I wouldn't be able to eat. I hadn't eaten very much since Sandy was back in the hospital, but I had been forcing myself to eat the bare minimum to keep up my strength. How could I eat knowing that Sandy would never eat again?

My husband had just died. This totally changed all of our lives drastically, yet life went on around us as if nothing had happened. The sky was blue, birds were singing, and children could be heard laughing and playing. How could things seem so normal when my husband just died? Sandy lived and died, and life went on as usual, as if he had never existed.

My parents and brother respected my silence during lunch, knowing that I had to deal with an awful lot.

Telling the children

After lunch, we went to the elementary school and then to the pre-school to pick up all the children. When the children entered the car, I acted as normal as possible and asked about their day. We made small talk, and not one of the children asked about their dad. I'm sure that they were afraid.

When we arrived at my parents' house, I told the children that I had to speak to them privately. We sat in a circle together on the floor in my old bedroom. This was the most difficult task that I have ever had to do in my life.

I began by saying, "We have to talk about Dad."

There was a pause, and then Jamie asked, "How is Dad?"

All of their sweet precious eyes were on me anxiously awaiting a positive answer.

I said, "Your daddy died this morning a little after 2:00. He was in such horrible pain, and the doctors did everything that they could for him. He is finally at peace. He's in Heaven now. He will always be watching over you as you do your best work in school, play your best games in soccer and baseball, and he will be up there watching you grow up into fine young men."

The boys all started to cry.

Adam then asked me in a choked up voice, to reenact exactly what happened when their dad died. I explained how he was having a horrible time gasping for air because his lungs were filling up with fluid. I explained that all of his organs stopped working due to the cancer, so he just couldn't stay alive. I told them how hard their dad fought to live, but it was agonizing, and now he was in peace.

Prompted by their requests, I lay down on the bed in the room and demonstrated how their dad was breathing and how he took his final breath. I told them that the moment their dad stopped breathing, I could just tell that he was no longer in his body. I explained my belief that his spirit had risen up out of his body, and his body appeared to be just an empty shell.

"Boys," I said, "I know that right now as I am speaking to you, Dad is watching over us."

I told them that I felt their dad's presence as I drove home from the hospital after he died. They seemed comforted by this.

My parents, listening in the background, came into the room and helped comfort their emotionally broken grandchildren. My little Jordan said, "You mean I'll never get to see my daddy again?"

"No," I told him, "But you will always keep the love and the memories of him in your heart and mind."

My poor children only four, six, and ten years old, lost their daddy. I couldn't believe that this could happen to us. They learned sorrow, hurt, and disappointment so much sooner than they should have.

Later that afternoon we met with Jim Kaufman to talk to the children and learn about Sandy Smith. Jim was wonderful with all of us. He explained the philosophy of death and was very comforting to us. He told us that although Sandy died, he continues to live on in all the boys and will live on in their children, and never be forgotten. He then gave each of the boys a piece of paper and pen and told them to write a goodbye letter to their dad. That night I prepared my own letter to be read at the funeral. I wanted everyone to know how bravely Sandy had tried to fight the cancer.

The boys completed their letters and as Jim read each one he started to cry. Jordan was too young to write, so he drew a great big "heart of love" for his daddy. Jamie and Adam's letters were so beautifully and sensitively written that both Jim and I felt that they should be read at the funeral. Part of me wishes that I still had the letters for keepsake, but they were buried with Sandy.

The copies that Jim read at the funeral were misplaced during that period of great upheaval and emotion.

That night, my parents took the four of us out for dinner, which I still couldn't eat. Adam asked me what I was going to do with his dad's clothes. I told him that I couldn't think about that for a while. Then he asked if I was going to take my wedding ring off. I told the boys that soon after the funeral I would remove my wedding ring, because by dying, their father had let me go. I would no longer be considered a married woman. I would now be referred to as a widow.

Between my mother and many of my friends, the word was circulated about when and where the funeral would be the next day.

It was agreed that the boys would stay with their grand-parents another night, because I had so much to do at home and at that time, I was not really emotionally equipped to take care of the children.

My friends told the elementary and pre-school that Sandy had passed away, and not to expect the children to be back in school until Monday.

Even though I was home alone that Wednesday night before the funeral, my friends Bettylou, Benay, and Carol, kept calling me regularly, each one of them wanting to come over and be with me. I told each of these wonderful, caring, friends, that I would be fine by myself. I really needed time to grieve alone.

Later that night there was a knock at my door. It was my neighbor, Richard. "Hi," he said. He handed me a piece of paper and said, "Here is the telephone number of the doctor at the Norris Cancer Center."

In my emotional state, I rather abruptly handed him back the paper and said, "It's too late, he died."

Richard was speechless, probably for the first time in his life. I just shut the door.

Around midnight, I was crying hysterically, as I took Peetie out for his late night walk. A few of my neighbors, who were out walking their dogs, came over to me, and I told them that Sandy had died. They were very kind and comforting. Later, they brought over food and flowers.

Exhausted, I finally got ready for bed and went to sleep

about 1:30 A.M. Suddenly I awoke to Sandy's voice calling to me. I heard him say, "Kath? Kath?"

I sat up in bed, my heart pounding. I said, "San? San? Is that you?" Peetie, who never stayed upstairs at night, was in my room panting excitedly and pacing around my bed. Peetie also seemed to sense Sandy's presence. I never heard any more. However, it was a little scary.

I spoke out loud to Sandy telling him that he would be laid to rest the next day. I cried and told him how much I loved him and how I missed him, and cried myself back to sleep.

The next morning, baskets and flowers started arriving.

The funeral

I pulled myself together, put on a black suit that Sandy had loved, and drove with my brother to the funeral.

We stopped at my parents' house and I helped the boys dress. They were unusually quiet, for good reason.

My parents and the boys followed behind me on the way to the mortuary. We parked and walked into the chapel. I was trying so hard to gain my composure.

Sheila, Alvyn, Randy, Pam, and her fiance', Scott, all arrived. We broke down into each other's arms.

Then the funeral director came over to me and said that the law required me to identify Sandy's body before the casket was closed. Gary tells me that he was never asked to identify *Kathie*, two years earlier. The casket was to be closed during the ceremony due to Sandy's request years before.

I went into the room and saw him lying in the casket that I had chosen, wearing the jogging suit that I had brought for him. It looked different with a shirt on underneath. I was crying as I told the director that he was my husband, Sanford Louis Smith.

I looked down at Sandy. He looked better than he had in the hospital. The makeup restored normal color to his face, so he wasn't so yellow. He actually had a slight smile on his lips. The scab which he received when he walked into the telephone pole while in Santa Monica with Adam was still on the side of his hand. That was less than a week ago. The scab hadn't even healed yet and Sandy was dead.

I put a rose, our goodbye letters, and photos of the family

in Sandy's hands. This man would be buried with a known history of all who loved him.

Sheila, Randy, and Pam then joined me. Sheila was hysterical. She also put a picture of herself in his casket, plus more flowers.

My mother called to me and told me that Adam was adamant about coming in to see Sandy. I said, "If he wants to, it's okay."

Adam walked up to his dad's casket and was practically at eye level with him. Without saying anything, he stood looking at his dad for a good three minutes, turned around, and silently walked out. I hoped that he would be okay.

As I walked out of the room, a very classy, flashy lady who had pulled up in a Rolls Royce, came over to me. Lee, was the client for whom Sandy had built the 16,000 square foot home for, in Bel Air. She had contacted my mother earlier and told her that as a tribute to Sandy she would cater the reception at my parents' home after the funeral. She said that she was ordering only the finest foods and food servers. She told my mother that none of us would have to lift a finger. We were so appreciative.

Lee approached me, hugged me, and said that she had arrived a bit early because she wanted to say goodbye to Sandy. He had been a good friend to her as well as her builder. I said okay, and let her into the room, although the casket had already been closed.

About ten minutes later, Lee came out with a smile on her face. She said that he was going to be fine. She claimed to be very spiritual and psychic and she believed that she could communicate with the dead.

Finally it was time for the funeral to begin. Many of my relatives had flown in from around the country to be there for me.

The boys, my parents, Sheila, Alvyn, Randy, Pam, Scott, Rick, and my nephew, Matthew, all sat with me in the private family section of the chapel. I was so touched by the tremendous turnout of friends who attended, since it was in the middle of a Thursday afternoon.

The service was beautiful, and Jim Kaufman read my farewell letter to Sandy along with the boys' letters. There wasn't a dry eye in the chapel. What a send off Sandy had.

Following the ceremony, friends and family came up to me and offered their love and support. I have been blessed with such wonderful people in my life.

Lee approached our family, obviously amused. She told us that Sandy's spirit was at the funeral. She said that she was laughing because Sandy had told her that he was surprised that there was such a large turnout of people there. We all stood there speechless. This felt eerie because that was a comment that Sandy would have made.

Lee then told me that Sandy must have fulfilled his purpose in this life and it was time for him to move on. I told her that I couldn't believe that his purpose had been fulfilled yet, because he was young and had three young children to help raise. She responded by telling me that perhaps he was just meant to father the children, but not meant to raise them as their father. She said that maybe he died prematurely to make me a stronger person or to teach me a lesson that I was meant to learn in my life. This spiritual outlook was very hard to hear at this time, and hard to believe.

Then we went to the gravesite that I had chosen, and Sandy was laid to rest. As his casket was lowered into the ground, everyone shoveled some dirt into the burial plot. Little Jordan saw this and cried out," Why is everybody pouring dirt all over my daddy?"

Again, almost everybody there broke down and wept. They wept for the premature loss of life. They wept for the broken woman who would be left alone to raise three small children. They wept for the three small children who lost their daddy.

This was not the way life was supposed to be.

Following the funeral, everyone came to my parents' house where Lee's catering crew served a magnificent meal.

It felt so good to be surrounded and embraced with so much love, including my aunts, uncles and cousins. My friends, Bettylou and Barry, Bob and Eileen, Bob and Janette, Candy and Marv, Carol and Marshall, Benay and Jeff, Morrie and Diane, Eve, Sylvia and Alan, Andrea and Mitch, Amy and Alan, Joni, Riva, Mira and Vic, and so many more, gave me the strength and hope to move on. Between my wonderful family and friends, I was never left alone unless I wanted to be alone.

The teachers from the boys' elementary and pre-school came to the funeral and sent beautiful baskets of food. We were a broken family, but we had a tremendous amount of support to sustain us.

While I was preparing for the funeral and arranging my finances with my father, my neighbor and friend, Graciella, walked our dog. A few weeks later, another neighbor paying a condolence call, asked me if I knew what happened to Graciella when she came into my townhouse to get Peetie. I didn't know anything. He told me that one late afternoon when Graciella entered my house, she grabbed the leash, and called for Peetie to come to her. When Peetie came to her, he was unusually restless. As she hooked the leash to his collar, she heard Sandy's voice from upstairs calling, "Kath? Kath?" Sound familiar?

Graciella, who was scared to death by this, answered, "No, Sandy, Kathy is not here. I, Graciella, have come to walk Peetie". She then quickly ran out of the door. This would not be the end of these strange occurrences.

After the funeral

I was overwhelmed with what needed to be done. It was amazing to me how much work was required to finalize financial affairs. Our finances were in complete disarray, with a great deal of credit card debt, as well as three mortgages on the old apartment building that I now solely owned.

The first thing that I had to do, was find Sandy's life insurance policies and collect on them. There wasn't a great deal to collect, since a year before, he had canceled a policy for another one with lower premiums. Thank God for my father's guidance and help. I could not have understood these complicated matters without him. Luckily, he had recently retired from his medical practice and was able to devote a tremendous amount of time helping me settle all of the affairs.

Settling the financial affairs

I completed the paperwork, and a couple of weeks later, a benefit arrived, made out to me in the amount of $10,000,000. I couldn't believe it! It was fairly late at night when I opened my mail, so when I saw this amount, I thought that I was hallucinating due to my tremendous stress. I called my father and said to him, "Daddy, I'm going to read you a number. Please tell me how much money it is."

So, I told him, and he said, "Why Honey, that is ten million dollars."

I told him that this was the benefit amount I had received from one of the insurance companies. Maybe that was where all the money had gone all these years, to pay a premium for a large insurance policy!

The insurance company had made a slight error, sending me someone else's claim and I was going to receive a small fraction of ten million dollars after all.

The other insurance policy took quite a while to collect because it was relatively new. The insurance company had to research the death claim thoroughly to rule out the suspicion that Sandy had been knowingly ill when he purchased the policy. Fortunately the insurance company came through and paid me, a few months later than expected.

Sandy had so much unfinished business and so much debt, that it took a tremendous amount of time, working daily with my father, to sort things out and pay all of the outstanding debts and bills. Unfortunately, paying off all the debt ate up a substantial amount of the life insurance money.

There was no way that I could have kept up with the Mercedes car payments, so I disposed of the car one month after Sandy died. My parents purchased a new Lexus and gave me their Toyota Cressida. They made a deal with the Lexus people to take the Mercedes and assume my payments.

I didn't make any money with this deal, but it relieved me of the astronomical payments, and it was one less obligation.

With mixed feelings, I turned the keys over to the Lexus dealership, and watched them drive the car over to their used car lot.

I felt sad that I had to give up the car, because Sandy had loved it so. This was just another affirmation that my life was changing and would never be the same.

Every day for a week, I drove past the Lexus used car lot to see my Mercedes. Then one day, it wasn't there anymore.

After giving up the Mercedes, it was time to think about

Sandy's Corvette. Immediately after he died, the body shop fixed the extensive damage caused by Sandy's accident. I couldn't afford to keep it. The insurance, alone, was more than I was financially able to handle.

My nephew, Randy, had a business associate who was interested in the Corvette, so I ended up selling him the car in November. Once again, I didn't make much on the sale, but it relieved me of a great responsibility.

Through my tears, I made the buyer promise to take good care of the car because it was one of Sandy's favorite possessions. I wept as he drove the car away.

Even though these cars were just materialistic possessions, with Sandy's passing they became more than just items. They were a part of him. He was gone, and now they were gone.

And then there was the old, unwanted apartment building. With my father's guidance, I used insurance money to pay off two mortgages, and was down to only one now.

When Sandy purchased the building he put very little money into it. He just landscaped a bit and threw a coat of paint on it. Right after he died everything seemed to go wrong. Seventy feet of gas line blew and I had to replace the pipes. A good portion of the roof had to be replaced. Then the Department of Building and Safety cited me for electrical deficiencies. If that weren't enough, the insurance company wouldn't reinsure the building until all of the cement walkways were replaced. All of this was costing me a fortune. There was still more. Because the apartment was still having leaking problems, gutters had to be installed around the whole building.

I couldn't keep up with all of the expenses, so I put the building up for sale. After inspection, I was informed that the furnaces in each of the units were non-functional. They had not been replaced since the building was built, more than fifty years earlier, another surprise expense. Sandy told me, knowing that I was upset about the purchase, that if he ever died, I could sell the building for a good profit. Wishful thinking. The real estate market was terrible at this time and a good sale didn't look too promising.

Eventually, I had to give the building back to the previous owner, who held the note. The building never did sell for my low asking price, and if I had dropped it lower, there would have been even more negative financial complications.

The previous owner was quite happy because I had made so many improvements to the building. When he took over owner-ship again, he turned around and sold the building dirt cheap, since he owned the building free and clear.

I was relieved, even though I lost quite a bit of money throughout the years.

Hospital bills

Adding to my aggravation, Cedars Sinai Hospital imme-diately began harassing me about Sandy's final hospital bill.

The hospital administrators knew about my medical in-surance coverage and they were paid very well, but they wanted the rest immediately. I told them that I would do my best. I was also furious because their bill reflected charges for oxygen the day after Sandy died. Rather than adjusting the bill, the hospital re-sponded by turning me over to their collection agency. Even San-dy's doctors tried in vain to help. The bottom line was, "Pay us the money now! No excuses!" The hospital had me in tears.

I was so outraged that I ended up screaming at the man who worked for the collection agency. I totally lost control over the phone, crying and screaming that I was in great financial dis-tress, having just been widowed with three children to support. "Give me a break!" I screamed, "I can't pay right now! You re-ceived the insurance money and the insurance will soon pay more of the balance!"

The man from collections just responded by telling me that the money was due NOW. I hung up on him. This was just too much to deal with all at once.

I was strong through this continual onslaught; although, there were times when the reality of everything would come crash-ing down on me and I would break down.

Working through the hospital mess was a job that took months to clear. Everything was a hassle.

Managing the days

While going through these challenging times, I still main-tained my property management position and carried out my responsibilities fully. I never told my boss what I was going through, even though he was a sensitive man and probably sensed my pain.

Maintaining the children's life style was more important than ever. I took the children to school every day, and I made sure that they never missed their soccer and baseball practices. The weekends were filled with their soccer or baseball games. I even continued as the Team Mom for their teams.

Adam's team, the team that Sandy was to coach, donated money to the soccer organization "...in memory of their coach, Sandy Smith." I was very touched by this gesture. The American Youth Soccer Organization could not have been more wonderful, sensitive, and supportive to our family.

Social Security Death Benefits did help the children. This monthly payment plus my property management job made it possible to stay where I was living, modest that it was, and support the children on my own.

A visit to the cemetery

Sandy was buried on a Thursday. I took the boys to a birthday party the following Sunday. It was only three days since the funeral, but I wanted the boys to get back in their routines and "live" again. The party wasn't far from the cemetery, so I told the boys that I wanted to visit Dad's grave to see how it looked with grass covering it.

As we drove there, Jamie became very upset telling me that it was stupid to go to the cemetery. Dad was dead and gone. He told me that I should stop crying and get on with my life.

I told Jamie that it was okay to grieve. I was sad and I wasn't going to hide it. In time I would get better, but now I needed to cry. I needed to visit the cemetery. Jamie had not cried openly since I told him of his father's death.

When we got to the cemetery, Jamie opted to stay in the car. It was okay. Adam, Jordan, and I walked over to the grave and put some flowers down. We cried together, and then Adam, always my most inquisitive child, said, "Mom, you know how Dad is in the box wearing his jogging suit?"

I sad, "Yes."

"Well...Is he naked up in Heaven?"

I began to laugh between my tears. What a question. I told

him that his dad was probably wearing a robe or something. I didn't think that he was naked.

Around mid-November, the weather began to get much cooler and it started to rain. I was very restless and uneasy thinking of Sandy in a wet, cold grave. It was one of the most unsettling feelings that I had ever had, and I continued to feel this for the first few years following his death. It was hard to come to terms with the reality of his death without feeling discomfort.

Unexplainable events

A few days later, I came home after having been gone all day. Sandy's cologne was permeating my bedroom so strongly that I thought for sure it had all spilled. I went over to the cabinet where it was still kept, and was shocked to see the bottle perfectly upright and sealed tightly. I picked the bottle up and smelled it, and there was no odor. Yet still, the essence filled the room. I then looked up and said, "Sandy, you must be here."

Then the telephone rang, and I left the room to take the call. When I returned to the room fifteen minutes later, the odor was completely gone. It really felt like Sandy had been there.

Another strange occurrence happened one night when I got into bed. I straightened my legs under the covers, and one spot at the foot of my bed was very warm, as if someone had been sitting there. Yet no one had been in the room. I moved my feet over to feel the rest of the bed, and it was cold, except for the one spot. Who can explain it? I do believe that it was Sandy, once again watching over me. It couldn't have been Peetie, the dog, because he had been asleep downstairs for the entire evening, and it couldn't have been the boys because they were asleep.

As time passed, these strange occurrences happened less frequently.

The children go on

On a positive note, Jamie was very busy, having been cast as the voice of Charlie Brown the year before. He was making commercials, a TV special, and he was in the first Charlie Brown Christmas special made in twenty years. We were so proud of him. I'm glad that Sandy was alive for part of this excitement. Coincidentally, Jamie was hired to be Charlie Brown for an American Lung Association public service announcement. How appropriate after what he had just experienced with his dad.

The boys and I were in the car on our return from one of Jamie's Hollywood auditions. It was raining and hailing, and we were stuck in bumper-to-bumper traffic on the Hollywood Freeway. All of a sudden Adam said, "Mom, it smells like Dad back here."

I was puzzled by his remark and asked him what he meant.

"You know, it smells like Dad when he was in the coffin," he said.

Evidently he must have smelled some chemical odor that reminded him of formaldehyde. I just explained to him that the rain and dampness sometimes makes different odors.

A few days later I was in the car with Jordan and he was in quite a talkative mood. Jordan is also very sensitive and could sense from my expressions when I was thinking of his dad. He would just look at me sometimes and say, "It's Dad, right?" I would tell him that he was right.

One day we were driving and Jordan said, "Momma, don't worry because I think that we can bring Dad back to us."

"How do you think that could happen?" I asked.

Jordan answered, "Well, I saw just last week in a movie where this guy died like Dad. A little while later some men took the dirt off of his grave and opened the box and the guy came out! Mom, are Dad's eyes open or closed in the box?"

I answered that they were closed.

Jordan then said, "Oh, well that could be a problem. But anyway, let's have those men that put the dirt on Dad, come back and take the dirt off of him, and then he can push the box open with his hands, and come out!" Jordan than demonstrated with his hands how his dad could push the coffin open.

This thought of Jordan's was so precious that I hated to tell him the truth. I told him that this idea worked well in the movies because movies could make things up that really couldn't happen in real life, and that in real life when someone died and was buried, there was no way that they could ever come back to life. I reminded my little four year old again that the doctors had done everything that they could to keep his dad alive but he was so sick and in so much pain, that he had to die. There was no way that he could ever come back to life.

Jordan suddenly became very quiet and then he said, "Momma, I remember Dad's face, but I'm starting not to remember how his voice sounded."

I told him that I felt the same way, but we at least had our memories of him and we had lots of pictures to help us remember.

Adam's second grade teacher told me that she felt that Adam was expressing much of his grief in his artwork. All of his paintings and drawings were black or very dark. Oh, my poor children.

As each year passed, the children asked about their dad's degree of decomposition. They wanted to know if he was a skeleton yet, if his eyes were still there, if he was dirty, and if there were bugs in the coffin with him. I was straightforward with them, although I made it clear that I was not an expert in pathology. They seemed satisfied with my explanations. They are quite inquisitive. I also felt a great satisfaction that they could open up and communicate these uncomfortable issues with me.

I saw the hurt, frustration and anger in my children and for a few years sought the help of several social workers and psychologists.

I was so angry with Sandy for dying and ruining our lives and I felt profound sadness that he would never see his boys grow up or share in the happiness of milestones yet to come. I was also feeling terribly lonesome. It was time to get into the support group.

The support group

Six weeks after Sandy's death, I received a questionnaire from the Hospice Program, asking how I was managing emotionally. I promptly responded, letting them know that I was not doing well emotionally and I was very depressed and stressed to the max. This six-week period had been pure hell, paying off debts, canceling Sandy's twenty-some credit cards, dealing with the hospital administration, and more. It also wasn't easy raising three little boys who had just lost their dad.

Surprisingly, Hospice contacted me quickly after receiving my questionnaire. They gave me the names of some support groups, one of them being specifically for young widows and widowers. I knew that this was the group for me. My friends and family were wonderful and very supportive, but they still didn't know what it was like to actually live my situation.

I decided to call. While I was waiting for her return call, I started to reflect on the past eight weeks since Sandy died.

Jo-Ann Lautman, the facilitator of the support group for young widows and widowers, returned my call. She was warm and comforting, and although I was apprehensive about joining a group, she put me at ease.

After hearing my story, she placed me in the group for newly widowed people. She was running three groups. The second group was for those who had dealt with the initial grief and now needed support learning to live alone again. The third group, Transition, consisted of widows and widowers ready to go on with their lives and perhaps begin dating again. I couldn't imagine ever making it to the third group.

I joined the group in November, which was the following month. We met every other Tuesday evening from 7:00 to 9:00.

About a week before the first support group meeting, I received a memorable call. It was from Pam Ogus, another widow in the group. Jo-Ann had told the group about my loss and that I would be coming to the next meeting.

Pam introduced herself, and told me that after hearing my story she felt compelled to call me. She said that she really related to me because her husband also had cancer, but he had suffered greatly for ten years. He had been Sandy's age and Pam was left with two boys. She was my first contact with someone who could really understand, having gone through this herself. I was so comforted by her phone call. I was deeply touched that she extended her love and support to me when she was so burdened with grief herself.

Pam told me that she would come by my house and pick me up so that we could attend the support group together. I was so happy and so relieved to have her support and company because I was very apprehensive.

Marta, my housekeeper, came that Tuesday night to babysit the children while I was at the support group.

Pam picked me up as planned, and when we met, I felt as

if we had been friends our whole lives. She is still one of my dearest friends.

When we arrived at the support group, Jo-Ann introduced herself and then we entered the room. I was pleasantly surprised by the setting of the room. It was like anybody's living room. There were two over sized sofas, two easy chairs, and about seven free-standing chairs, all set up around a coffee table with coffee, tea, and some dessert and candy. The room was warmly lit by the lamps on the end tables. I was grateful that the large overhead fluorescent lights were not used. The room was warm and cozy, and made one feel comfortable and at ease.

Sitting next to Jo-Ann, I looked at the other people. I couldn't believe that all these people were in "the same place" that I was.

There were about ten women and only one man there that day, all approximately my age. Jo-Ann started the support group meeting by introducing me. Then she asked me to tell the group the story of my loss. I thought that I would be really nervous, speaking to a group of strangers, but as soon as I began telling my story, the other people nodded their heads and cried along with me. This was where I belonged. These people could really understand my feelings because they were living the same nightmare.

After I finished, the others shared the stories of their losses, and then people talked about grief issues that they were currently experiencing. Towards the end of the session, Jo-Ann read some beautiful poetry, and she gave us each a copy. Then she ended the group, as she would each session, with words of encouragement and understanding. Everyone in the room hugged each other. We were bound together by tragedy.

I couldn't wait until the next session. It felt as if a weight was slowly releasing itself from my heart.

My thirty-ninth birthday was in October. My friends, Eileen and Janette, saw to it that I wasn't alone. They picked me up in the late morning, took me for a make-over, bought me the makeup, and took me out to lunch. They helped to make a very difficult day very special.

A bad moment

Following my lunch, I picked the boys up from school and

rushed Adam to the field for his soccer practice. We waited for twenty minutes, but no one showed up. Practice had been canceled. I had neglected to listen to my answering machine in my hurry to get him to practice.

Adam, only seven, was upset and started to cry. Then he jumped out of the car and ran down a nearby residential street. Jamie, Jordan, and I jumped out of the car to run after him, but he had vanished. We quickly got back into the car and slowly drove in the direction where we saw him run. We drove around the neighborhood three times, and then went back and searched the whole soccer field. Adam was nowhere to be found. I started to panic. Jamie started crying, saying that his brother was gone for good.

We drove up and down Van Nuys Blvd., and then went back to the neighborhood to search again. There was still no sign of him. Finally, I drove a couple of miles up to Ventura Blvd. It didn't seem likely that he would go so far away, but what other choice did I have? I just couldn't believe that this was all happening. How much more could I handle before totally breaking down?

Thankfully, up at Ventura Blvd., Jamie screamed out, "There he is! There he is!"

Adam was running down the street hysterically crying. I honked my horn, and when he saw us, I motioned for him to stay where he was while I turned the car around.

When we caught up with him, we were all crying. He told us that he had stopped at a gas station, borrowed some money, and called home, but we weren't there. Then he said that he was looking for the freeway to walk home.

Oh God, I couldn't believe it. Thankfully, my troubled little boy was safe with me again, and we drove home.

I was an emotional basket case, having lost my husband, and almost a child. I broke down and started to cry again. Pam, my wonderful widow friend, called me and she helped me pull myself back together.

"Alone" with friends

That evening, Marta came to babysit, because two couples, Eileen, Bob, Janette, and her Bob, were taking me out for a birthday dinner. They had done so much for me already, but wanted to do more.

Eileen and Bob picked me up and we all went to a lovely restaurant in Studio City. This was the first time that I was out with other couples since Sandy died. We were seated at a table for six, yet there were only five of us. I was acutely aware of the empty seat beside me. It would take a while to get used to being the "odd" one at the table when I was out with friends. Coincidentally, Gary's first outing as a widower was at the same restaurant. He was also the odd number at his table, experiencing the same feelings.

This evening was especially difficult for me. I felt terribly lonely. I missed being a couple. The episode with Adam earlier that day made me more emotionally vulnerable. When the evening was over, I came home and cried myself to sleep, wondering how I could face another day.

Our grief management - a beginning

The days began to go by more easily. The children were into their routines, and I was starting to socialize with my friends again. Most of the financial affairs were now in order. My property management job was going well and my boss was satisfied with my work. Finally I was able to relax a bit and have some leisure time.

I was surfacing from the ordeal of tragedy and loss, as a stronger and more independent woman. I was no longer afraid to be alone or to raise my children alone. I was managing things well, developing my confidence again, and proving Sandy wrong. He had worn down my self-esteem for so long, that I doubted that I could survive without him. I was a grieving widow, yet I felt relief from his emotional and verbal abuse.

Some people have asked why I have experienced grief, since I was often treated so poorly. I did love him. I felt badly that the children had to go through such a traumatic event, and I missed and craved the positive traits that Sandy brought to our relationship. I felt loss and grief. I was lonely without a partner, and I felt the loss of a relationship, which always had the potential to get better. I was reacting to the abrupt change in my life. Some other members of the support group were also in less than ideal marriages, and they also felt significant loss.

I saw my wonderfully supportive friends, Bettylou, Ronna, and Rhoda every day at the elementary school. We were referred to as "The Girls" because we were always together. We are still like sisters, and our children are friendly too. The girls lived through every experience with me and they were there to comfort me and give whatever support I needed. We would meet for breakfast, coffee, or lunch, occasionally combined with shopping. Bettylou would even make the rounds with me on my job, or she would accompany me to my old, decrepit Hollywood apartment building. Besides my family, she was my strongest support during that time. Bettylou understood my feelings, because she lost her only sibling to cancer. She still hasn't recovered from her grief. When I would cry over Sandy, she would cry along with me, while acknowledging the contrasts between a sibling and a husband.

The Widow Pam, as she would come to be known, was also there for me, as I was for her. We still spoke every night. It helped pass the loneliness of the late evenings when the grief over our losses became so acute.

I distinguish her as The Widow Pam because of my niece named Pam. I always referred to her as The Widow so my friends would know which Pam I was referring to. Soon everyone who was close to me referred to Pam as The Widow Pam. In time, Pam would also introduce herself to my friends as The Widow. This may sound strange to someone unfamiliar with the people involved, but it was always taken as a loving and humorous, if a little ironic, gesture.

I continued to look forward to the support group. Many sessions introduced at least one new person. At first, there were only women. I think most of us were a little relieved when the balance began to even out, since it was closer to the real world in which we were trying to recover our ground.

December 5, 1991 would have been Sandy's 45th birthday. The boys and I lit one candle in his memory. I explained to the boys that we were not lighting candles to celebrate Dad's birthday, but we were lighting the one candle to celebrate that their dad once lived and still lived on in our hearts.

When Jamie and I were alone, I noticed him looking at the lit candle. When I asked him what he was thinking, he spoke in a very shaky voice, "I get this horrible feeling in my stomach when I think about Dad."

I explained to him that this was a symptom of his feeling grief, that it was okay to cry, and doing so would probably help him to feel better. He told me that he was unable to cry. He has finally started to deal with his grief within the past five years.

Soon after this conversation, something very shocking occurred, involving Jamie, then age ten, and a classmate in school. Jamie was in his physical education class, and he and a classmate started to argue over something. The argument had escalated rapidly and became physical when the fellow classmate accused Jamie of causing his father's death. Jamie went into such intense rage, that it took four large teenage boys to pull him off of the classmate. Children can be so insensitive and hurtful. A school administrator told me what happened. Jamie never said a word. Life wasn't getting easier for these poor bereaved children.

Through my support group, I found out about a grief group for children, ages seven to fourteen years. This group, meeting for six consecutive weeks, was sponsored by the Big Brothers and, conveniently, it was held in the same place as my support group, led by two social workers. I immediately enrolled both Jamie and Adam for the March session. Jordan was still too young. I could hardly wait for the group to begin. The children really needed to be among other children who had experienced the same loss.

I meet Gary

December 18, 1991, the bereavement groups united for a holiday party. I was nervous because the party involved all three widow and widower support groups, which included people farther along in their grief process than I.

The Widow Pam and I attended this party together. When we arrived, I was amazed by how many people were there. Pam introduced a girlfriend of hers, named Gail. Gail was in the advanced Transition group having lost her husband suddenly, of a heart attack two years earlier. Gail then introduced us to Jill, whose husband had died two years before from cancer. These girls would end up being very good friends of mine.

Jo-Ann then rearranged everyone into smaller groups. Pam and I were placed in separate groups. When I walked over to my assigned group area, the most adorable, handsome man was sitting there. It was the first time that I started to spark feelings for a man again. I was surprisingly disappointed and even a little jealous that this beautiful man was massaging another widow's neck. They seemed very close to one another, and I assumed that they were dating.

When we began our little group, the man introduced himself as Gary Young. He told us that his wife had died of breast cancer two years earlier, and that he was in the Transition group. He was so warm and sensitive. I knew that this was the kind of man I wanted. The widow receiving the neck massage introduced herself as Anna. Her husband had died three weeks before the birth of her second child. She was also in the Transition group.

I enjoyed this evening and hoped to see some of these people again. It helped to see how people healed within a two-year period. I hoped that I would get there one day. I thought about Gary Young. Boy, that Anna was lucky.

Chapter 13: DATING

My first spark

Our grief group resumed after a two-week New Year hiatus. To my surprise, a man entered our group of ten women. The widows perked up immediately when they saw him, especially Jan. I could tell that she was already planning their future.

As usual, we took turns telling about our losses, as we did when new members entered the group. When it came to the man's turn, he introduced himself as **Jeff**. He certainly wasn't what you would call attractive, but he seemed quite sensitive and he moved me deeply when he spoke of his wife. He was an anesthesiologist and she had been a C.P.A. They had four children. His wife had been fighting cancer for over four years, and had passed away in December. To add to all of this, Jeff's father was critically ill and wasn't expected to live much longer. I really felt for him.

After group, I was shocked when Jeff approached me and told me how moved he was by my story. He then walked me out to my car, we wished each other well, and Pam and I drove home.

A few days later, I received a call from Jo-Ann telling me that Jeff's father had passed away. She felt that it was important for the group members to call him and offer support. I immediately called and left a message explaining to him who I was, and left my number in case he wanted to talk.

Three days later, much to my surprise, Jeff called me back. He told me that he really appreciated my call and we continued to talk for about an hour. We finally got on to the subject of movies. He said that he really enjoyed going to movies and often went by himself to escape the reality of what was going on in his life. I lightheartedly mentioned that I would join him sometime if he liked. He immediately asked me out, and we decided to go to the movies the following Saturday night. He would drive from his home in Santa Monica and pick me up at around 7:00. This would be my first outing with a man since Sandy died.

On Saturday, Marta came to babysit, and Jeff picked me up as scheduled. He won me over with his pleasant personality and apparent sensitivity. We chose the movie, "Grand Canyon," which had just opened. The movie happened to be filmed predominantly in Santa Monica where Jeff lived.

In one scene, they showed the Santa Monica Hospital. Jeff leaned over and whispered to me that his wife had died there. I reached over and patted his arm, offering comfort. When I attempted to pull my hand away, he grabbed it and held it against him. He didn't let go of my hand for the rest of the movie. My mind was racing. Did he want more than friendship? I just didn't know what to think. Being touched again really felt good. It had been a long time.

After the movie, Jeff continued to hold my hand as we walked to the car. We then drove to an Italian restaurant for a bite to eat.

During our dinner Jeff asked me questions about Sandy and he reached across the table and put his hand over my hand, offering me comfort. I thought he was the kindest man in the world.

After dinner, Jeff drove me home, kissed me good night, and he immediately asked me out for the following Saturday night. He told me to dress warmly, but he wouldn't tell me where we were going to go. He said it was a surprise.

I was on cloud nine. It felt so wonderful to be in the company of a man again, to be touched and be treated affectionately. I was starving for all of this.

When I arrived home, the children were up waiting for me. They wanted to know all about our evening. They thought that Jeff was really funny looking. They said that he looked like a mad scientist with his kinky, curly hair and bushy mustache. I told the boys that his looks didn't matter as long as he treated me well.

I wondered how the boys would react to knowing that I was going out with a man other than their father. To my relief, they were thrilled for me and they were excited to see me happy. I know that it does not always work out that way. They seemed relieved to see that I was finally going on with my life.

As I was getting ready for bed, I remembered that The Widow Pam was anxiously awaiting my call, telling her about my first date. She was thrilled for me and wanted to know every detail. As we were speaking, I was surprised to hear a "beep in" on my call waiting. Jeff had just arrived home and he called to thank me for a wonderful evening. This was so sweet of him. I was quickly becoming smitten.

As the week progressed, I could hardly wait for our next date. Bettylou, Ronna, and Rhoda were thrilled for me; and they were so wonderful, listening to me repeat my first date to them over and over again. They said that it was so good to see me "alive" again.

Finally Saturday arrived and I could hardly contain myself. My wonderful Marta came to babysit, as usual. She was also thrilled for me.

Jeff picked me up and told me that we would be stopping by his house. I said, "Oh, so you want to introduce your children to me."

"No," he replied. "The children are all out for the night."

He wanted to show me his house and have some champagne with me. It was a pleasure being in his company. He was so bright and stimulating.

When we arrived at his house, I was amazed. It was absolutely gorgeous. He took me on a tour and then showed me pictures of his children and his deceased wife. He then opened a bottle of champagne. We toasted to moving on in life, and proceeded to enjoy the bottle.

While we were drinking, Jeff showed me picture albums of his life and told me all about his family. The champagne was wonderful and I was getting a little tipsy because we hadn't eaten dinner yet. I wondered what he had in mind for dinner.

Suddenly, without notice, Jeff grabbed me and began to passionately kiss me. This was all going a little too fast for me. I was totally overwhelmed, and told him to slow down. He didn't want to. When I brought up to him that his wife was only gone a month, he replied by telling me that he knew she was dying for many months and he had been grieving for a long time. He was ready to move on and live again. I told him that I did not feel the same way, and that he should respect my feelings.

Then he took me to a nearby coffee shop for a bite to eat. I wasn't hungry anymore. My mind was in a whirlwind. We made small talk, and then he drove me home.

I called Bettylou and The Widow Pam, and told them what had happened. They told me to relax and have an enjoyable time.

I felt so much better after talking to them. Together with Ronna and Rhoda, they kept me afloat whenever I would start to sink. I was so lucky to have them in my life.

Jeff continued to call me late every night and we would talk for about an hour. We never really discussed what happened. He asked me out for the following Saturday night. This time he wanted me to drive to Santa Monica and we would go out from there. He said that the Valley was foreign to him and he felt more comfortable in Santa Monica. I agreed to drive out there and meet him at his house.

Jeff told me that he felt it was best to keep our relationship quiet and not let anyone in the group know. I agreed to this, although I felt that keeping secrets was foolish. But I also understood how it might be hard for some of the newer widows to hear about two members of the group dating.

As usual, The Widow Pam and I attended group together and although Jeff and I exchanged glances many times, our dating was kept secret. The Widow Pam knew, of course, and I had told Jo-Ann privately. She was delighted for us.

After group, Jeff walked me out to the parking lot. He told me that he had gone horseback riding at Griffith Park that day. I told him that Sandy was buried near there. He said that he remembered and he thought of him while riding. All of a sudden, I felt myself being pushed aside by Jan. She overheard Jeff telling me that he was horseback riding, so she jumped between us and said, "Oh Jeff, I love horseback riding! Why don't we go sometime? Are you free this weekend?"

Jeff was shocked, as was I. She was being very pushy, but of course, she did not know that Jeff and I were dating. Jeff regained his composure and told her that he was not available over the weekend. She continued to walk between us monopolizing the conversation. I met up with The Widow Pam and we drove home.

The following Saturday night I drove to Santa Monica, as planned. With favorable traffic, the trip can take forty-five minutes. We drove in Jeff's car to the Third Street Promenade, a festive outdoor mall with street performers. We had some drinks, and saw a movie. Then we returned to his house, he dismissed his sitter, and we settled down to watch TV.

Jeff's children were happy to meet me and seemed pleased that their father had a new friend.

After watching TV for a while, Jeff offered me a little wine. It was getting very late and I had a long drive ahead of me. He told me to sit with him and not to go yet. He promptly fell asleep, and I let myself out of his house and drove home. It was already around 2:30 A.M.

The next day, at about 2:00 in the afternoon, the boys and I went over to Jeff's house. All the children played, and then Jeff had dinner delivered. Even though we were invited as Jeff's guests, I ended up paying for our portion of the food. This wasn't right since he was much more financially secure than I, but I wasn't about to make a big deal over it.

After that weekend, Jeff continued to call me late every night and we would talk for hours. We would talk about his job, problems with nannies, and different crisis with the children. We seemed to be good for each other. Although, as time went on, I found that I was giving far more than I received.

Jeff continued to ask me out on the weekends, and he always expected me to drive to Santa Monica. Much to the disapproval of my parents and friends, I continued to make the drive weekly, always returning very late at night.

In late February, Jeff invited me to go to Palm Springs with him for a weekend. This sounded like great fun. It would be my first vacation since Sandy's death. Marta was able to babysit the boys from Friday through Sunday.

I didn't have such a great feeling about the weekend, sensing that Jeff was feeling pretty uncomfortable.

The day after we returned home, Jeff called me and said that we needed to have a talk. He asked me what I wanted out of our relationship. I told him that I was enjoying the companionship and friendship. He then told me that marriage was not something that was "in the cards" for him now or any time in the future. The obvious meaning behind his words was hurtful and very offensive. I was already less than satisfied by this relationship. He had become very selfish and self-centered. I was disappointed and offended that he thought I wanted marriage. It was much too soon to even consider a marriage.

He told me that he enjoyed my companionship, but that was all that he wanted.

I knew that it was time to move on.

Only days after this conversation, Patty, another widow in the group, called me because she was feeling very depressed and needed to talk with someone from group. She desperately wanted a man in her life and was feeling very frustrated and lonely. She asked me if I had started dating yet. I told her that I had been dating Jeff from our group since January. There was a long silence and then she told me something that would make me feel as if a dagger was forced into my heart.

She said, "You're dating Jeff?"

"Yes." I replied.

"Well", she said, "I was dating him too. About a month ago I asked him to accompany me to a formal affair, and he accepted. We then went out a few more times, and then he invited me and my girls over to his house and we all went to the beach. We even went to his daughter's birthday party."

All the time she was talking, I was shaking and in total disbelief. It's true that I would see Jeff perhaps once a week, but I couldn't believe that he would be dishonest about dating someone else, especially someone else in our group.

I was also hurt that he invited Patty and her children to his daughter's party. I had invited him and his children to Jordan's party. This was a slap in my face. Anyway, Patty went on to say that she thought that Jeff was going to marry her and "carry her into the sunset." She said he had been very attentive.

I was getting sicker by the minute.

She said, "He just suddenly stopped calling. I called him at his office, at his home, and he wouldn't even return my calls. That is why I am such a mess. So, if this was a contest, you won."

What a prize I got!

She said that their relationship had been totally platonic, although she wanted more. She claimed that her mental state was worse than ever because of the manner in which he rejected her.

That evening when Jeff called me I told him what Patty had told me, and that although we were not formally going steady, it was not morally or ethically right to play these secretive dating games with two widows in our group.

I begin to see a familiar pattern

Once again, the signs were all there, spelling out what kind of person he really was. But like a fool, I still continued to see him. If I had been stronger emotionally, I would have ended this hurtful relationship. I kept the relationship going only because I desperately needed to look forward to something. These weekend outings helped me through the lonely weeks. It was a relationship with escalating abuse, but at that time it felt comfortable and perhaps too familiar to me. I still had much emotional growth ahead of me.

He apologized for hurting me and he said that he just considered Patty a friend until she started becoming too demanding and getting on his nerves. He tried to make it up to me by taking me to dinner and to a concert. I still drove to his house first.

Jeff dropped out of the grief group after this incident, as he had hurt too many of us. Jo-Ann was angry when Patty told her what had happened, and she was very happy that Jeff had the good sense to stay away.

On a more positive note, this provided the incentive for me to start dating other people. I put the word out to all my friends.

The support group for children

That March, the children's grief group began. We reported to the same comfortable room where my grief group was held. All of the parents remained in that room, and the children were ushered into another room, equipped with tables, where they could write and do artwork.

Several parents from group were there with their children. I was thrilled to have The Widow Pam and her son, Adam, in the group. That beautiful man, Gary Young, who I had met that past

December, was there with his youngest daughter, Robyn.

The children's group was wonderful for them because they were among other children who had endured the loss of a parent, and very healing because there was a genuine outlet for anger, frustration, confusion, and loneliness. The children expressed themselves through art, culminating in a beautiful book compiled individually by each child, saying goodbye to their dead parent, each in their own way. These precious books will be cherished for a lifetime.

The Big Brothers Program

The children's grief group opened up a whole new avenue for my boys. The group facilitator was very taken by the boys and encouraged me to enroll them in the Big Brothers program. It could be a long process, so I wasted no time. The social worker interviewed the boys and cautioned us that the number of big brothers was not great, but touched by our story, she promised top priority. The boys met with her weekly for at least six weeks so that she could really get to know them in order to make proper matches.

Mary came through for us, and the boys were matched with the most wonderful, special men, Sheldon Levitt, Thierry Benchetrit, and Peter Swarth. Jamie and Adam were placed immediately and Jordan, who was only four years old at the time, was required to wait until he was six. Each of the boys remains close with their big brothers, after nearly a decade.

With full lives of their own, these wonderful, selfless men have made the time to present positive role models for the boys, and have voluntarily taken on the tremendous task of contributing to their emotional health. They have never expected anything in return for all the wonderful things that they have done and still continue to do.

Our neighbor, Alan Kopp, also offered unconditional comfort and support and is like another big brother to each of the boys. He continues to enrich our lives with his goodness, his generosity, and his many talents.

Getting to know Gary

The children's grief group enabled me to get to know Gary

better. He was terrific. The Widow Pam kept telling me that she sensed real chemistry between us, but I told her that she was imagining things. He had a steady girlfriend, who was not the widow, Anna, as I had suspected. Everyone felt that his girlfriend, Carla, a divorcee, was distant and uninteresting. I wondered what such a fabulous, vivacious, handsome guy was doing with someone like her. In a social setting, she was extremely quiet and withdrawn. Gary always did all of the socializing.

Gary and I became really good, close friends and I adored him. We met occasionally for completely platonic lunches. Sensing our mutual chemistry, he told me that the two of us could never end up together, nor even date, because the thought of handling three boys as aggressive as mine thoroughly overwhelmed him, especially since his experience had only been with daughters. I accepted his explanation and we continued to be the best of friends, always confiding in each other.

We often complained to each other about our problems with Jeff and Carla.

Gary fixed me up with Carla's cousin, an accountant, who was also widowed. He had just moved to California from the east, after losing his wife a few years earlier. I agreed to go out with him, while still seeing Jeff usually once a week, now on a more casual basis.

Ron certainly wasn't my "Prince Charming," but he was a nice guy. He was turning fifty, but acted much older, and like me, he was extremely needy. But he needed much more than I could give. I wanted to like him, but there just wasn't any chemistry with this troubled man. He was anxious to get me into bed, and he wanted to escalate the relationship far too quickly for me, which threatened my vulnerability. He did take me to the opera, to dinners, and to the movies, which was very generous of him but I never enjoyed his company. After dating for about a month, we mutually ended the brief relationship.

Ron also joined the grief group. After two sessions he quit the group, saying that it wasn't the right thing for him, but he did meet another widow, Cindy, and they began a full relationship. I was happy for both of them. She was a psychologist and he had problems. A match made in Heaven!

June was approaching and I knew that Father's Day might

be difficult for Jeff and his children. Jeff did not think of my children or me on Mother's Day. I never seemed to stand up for myself in this relationship, and I was too insecure to speak up most of the time, for fear of losing him and being alone again. Once again, I had become stuck in an abusive relationship.

I told Jeff that I would come out to Santa Monica one afternoon and take his children shopping for his Father's Day gifts. He said that would be fine, and he asked me to also pick out a birthday present from his girls to his son for his son's coming birthday.

I took the children shopping as planned, and then left Jeff with the receipts to reimburse me for the purchases. He took this act of generosity for granted and I never received one cent of reimbursement, even though I did not have much money, and he could well afford the cost. That was the last time I volunteered to go out of my way to do special things for his family.

And yet, I continued seeing Jeff one night every weekend. Soon my friends, knowing that I wanted to meet a nice guy, started coming through for me.

My friend, Faith, had a friend named **Brant**, a divorced man with two children. We met for lunch at Jerry's Deli in Encino. It was quite nerve-racking because I didn't know what he would look like. I arrived first and waited anxiously around the entrance to the deli, with mixed feelings as men of every description passed me. Then, there he was. True to Faith's description, he was very tall, lean, and quite handsome. He looked at me as he walked in and I looked at him and I said, "Brant?"

He responded with, "That's me!"

He made me feel good immediately when he told me how pretty he thought I was. He was very sweet and warm, and I found him quite talkative. It was quite a welcomed relief after being with uptight Jeff and disturbed Ron. Brant wasn't brilliant, but he was fun, and I liked him instantly.

After lunch he asked me to go along with him to pick up his bicycle at a local bike shop. He was very active in sports. He belonged to a bicycle club for Singles, and he was president of a local ski club for Singles. He also loved ice-skating, hockey, and roller-blading, like a big kid living through his second childhood. He was so warm and affectionate, like a big cuddly teddy bear.

He asked me out to dinner and to a L.A. Kings hockey game. Then he took me ice-skating with his friends.

My fortieth birthday

It was October of 1992, and I was turning forty years old. My brother, Rick, and my parents, decided to throw me a fortieth birthday party at Rick's house. I was in a real dilemma. Which man would I invite to accompany me to my party? I wasn't seeing Ron anymore, so that was one less to worry about. Now it was between Jeff and Brant. I decided to go ahead and ask Jeff, since I had just begun dating Brant.

I wasn't very optimistic that Jeff would agree to come to my party because he seemed to shy away from knowing anybody in my life. Much to my surprise, Jeff accepted the invitation and actually said that it would be his pleasure to be there. I felt that I had made the right decision. Perhaps there was hope after all.

Sweet Brant, not knowing about my party, invited me out to dinner for my birthday. I told him that I was busy on my birthday but would love to go out any other time. We decided on the Monday night following my birthday.

There were over sixty people on my guest list, and they all came, including Gary and his girlfriend. I was thrilled that Gary was coming since he was also invited to another party that he had previously accepted. He said that he would come to my party first, stay for a while, and then go on to the other party.

On the day of my party Jeff actually came to my place and picked me up. This was the first time that he had come to pick me up in months.

My party turned out more wonderful than I could ever have imagined. Rick had the house decorated with pink balloons and delicious hors d'oeuvres were served, followed by a magnificent buffet dinner. My father served marvelous champagne and red and white wine were served during dinner.

I was very moved when my father served everyone champagne and then made a beautiful toast to me. Everyone cheered and I was so happy. It was then my turn to make a toast to all of my wonderful friends and family. I thanked everyone for their support and love throughout my difficult period. I told all of them how much I loved them and that they made me rich, for their friendship was like gold to me. Everyone cheered, cried, and joyfully laughed, for how far I had come in a year. Gary tells me that he was impressed and perhaps a little envious that I had such a large circle of trusted friends. He tells me that he liked these people immediately, and hoped that one day he could somehow become part of that group.

Jeff was very anti-social, only speaking to those who first spoke to him. He lingered in the background, which was quite embarrassing to me. It was plain to see that he was very uncomfortable and really didn't want to be there.

I was ecstatic when Gary Young and his girlfriend arrived at the party. Whenever Gary was with me, I would feel this tremendous blanket of warmth and well-being. I was already falling in love with him.

Gary couldn't stay long, but had already made a wonderful impression on my family and friends.

After all of my guests left the party, I sat down with my family to open up my beautiful gifts. Jeff sat next to me, uneasiness emanating from him. When the opening of the gifts was completed, I waited to see Jeff's gift. He didn't say a word about a gift. He drove me home and asked if I would come over to his house the next night. Foolishly, as always, I agreed.

The next morning, my neighbor and good friend, Alan, came over to give me some of my gifts, which he had graciously transported home for me. I happened to mention to Alan that Jeff was the only one who didn't give me a birthday gift. Alan said that was strange because Jeff had told Alan that my gift from him was in his car. Go figure.

The next night, I drove to Jeff's, as usual. I must add that throughout this relationship, Jeff never offered to help me out with babysitting costs. In fact, on several occasions, I lent him money to pay his sitters when he didn't have the cash, and he never had the decency to pay me back. I was too uncomfortable to ask him for the reimbursement.

Jeff continued to hurt me, or better said, I let myself get hurt. I would find out that he went to a concert or to other affairs, excluding me, except on rare occasions. He treated me as if I were his secret mistress. Whenever I would ever question him about where he went, he would always be very evasive and say that he was out with friends.

I was totally unfamiliar with this type of treatment and naive enough that I didn't know how to deal with it.

Well, the tables turned when I started to date others. Sometimes when he would call, I was out on a date, or just leaving for one. He would have the audacity to ask me where I was going and with whom I was going. I gave him his own treatment, saying that I was going out with a friend. One time he asked me specifically if the friend was a man or a woman. I paused, enjoying this greatly, and said, "It's a friend."

I could actually detect a bit of jealously. He didn't really want me, but he certainly liked me to be there when he needed me to listen to his troubles. There were times when Jeff would pour out his heart to me for an hour. I would offer my thoughts and then go on to a few of my own problems. I would ask him a question, only to hear snoring as his only response. This was symbolic of the way our relationship had been going.

The night after my party, at Jeff's house, while watching TV, I asked him if he had a birthday present for me.

He responded by saying, " Yes. Do you want it now?"

What a weirdo!

Feeling pretty low, I told him that it would be very nice to have it since it was my birthday. I was surprised when the gift was a beautiful Liz Claiborne blouse with Indian beadwork.

Father's Day, 1992

As Father's Day, 1992 approached, I was becoming very sad and depressed again. It would be our first Father's Day since Sandy's death. Sheila's daughter, Pam, was going to be married that day. It was a very emotional time for all of us.

Two upsetting things occurred shortly before Father's Day. First, Sheila called me, and as politely as possible, asked me to return any items that had belonged to her and Sandy's parents. I told her that I didn't have much, but the few items that I had, I wanted to pass down from Sandy to my children.

I understood Sheila's point of view. She had lost both of her parents and her brother and desperately wanted to hang on to the things that brought back memories. However, my children were entitled to have something from their father's past. Weighing the importance of this situation in my mind, I came to the conclusion that Sheila should have the items since they meant such a great deal to her. She had gone through so much with these family losses, and this was something that I could do for her to help lessen her grief.

Prior to the wedding on Father's Day, we drove out to the cemetery to visit Sandy's grave. The boys brought the Father's Day gifts that they had made in school and placed them on their dad's grave. Jordan lay down on the grave and screamed towards the ground as loudly as he could, "I love you, Daddy! Happy Father's Day."

People visiting graves nearby started to cry when they saw and heard Jordan. I cried too. Jamie was silent. Adam asked to be left alone at the grave for a few minutes. Afterwards, we drove home and prepared for the wedding.

The boys were all included in the wedding ceremony so they had to wear tuxedos. Dressing them and myself took a bit longer than planned. Because we were in a hurry, I took what I needed out of my purse, dropped the purse on the dining room floor to pick up later, and we left for the wedding.

Pam's wedding was beautiful. Sandy would have been so happy. He should have been there. His presence was greatly missed by all that night.

We arrived home after the wedding around 11:30 P.M. When we came into the house, I went over to my cordless phone to call my parents to let them know that we arrived home safely. Then I saw the second upsetting incident for the day. The phone was gone, and so was my purse. I was very upset knowing that someone had been in my house. When the police arrived, they found that someone had entered through my patio sliding door. The strange part of this was that the only things that were missing were my cordless phone and my purse with all of my credit cards in it. The police helped me put a stick in the slider of the door for security, and the next day the landlord installed high security locks on all the doors.

I was an emotional mess that whole day, feeling like I was ready to go over the deep end. I had a very unsettled feeling in my stomach, knowing that someone had been watching us, but we didn't know who, when or for how long. When I called Jeff that night he was very distant and unsympathetic. He just didn't care.

The one-year anniversary

It seemed slow in coming and yet at the same time, in a strange way the events also seemed to go by blazingly fast, but August was soon approaching, with the one-year anniversary of Sandy's death. It was time to place a permanent headstone on the grave. Up to this point, I hadn't been ready to deal with the finality of his death. Now it was time to think about ordering Sandy's headstone and a decision had to be made if a formal unveiling ceremony would take place. I concluded that such a ceremony would be too painful for our children.

One day, in the middle of July, I went to the cemetery to order Sandy's headstone. Upon entering the building, an elderly gentleman approached me and asked what he could do for me. I told him that I was there to order my husband's head-stone. The gentleman looked at me in surprise and said, "You are much too young to be here ordering your husband's gravestone!"

When he said that, I started to cry. He was right. I shouldn't be here at all. Sandy should still be alive enjoying his life with his wife and children.

I gathered my composure and went about the task of ordering the headstone and choosing what it would say. The headstone simply read:

> **Sanford Louis Smith**
> **December 5, 1946 - August 27, 1991**
> **Beloved husband, daddy, and brother**

Sandy's headstone was ready by the first anniversary of his death. The boys and I went to the cemetery to see it. We were very quiet, immersed in our own thoughts.

The strange world of dating

As Christmas, 1992 arrived, Brant invited me to a Christmas Ski Club party. The party was fun, and it was a pleasure being out with a man who wasn't embarrassed to introduce me to his friends.

Brant was always very pleasant, but he was very much a

"Good Time Charlie." He had his own property management company, but was able to let others run it most of the time. This enabled him to enjoy his sports and hobbies whenever he wanted, so he was hardly ever in town. He asked me to join him on many occasions, but I had three children who could not be left alone. He enjoyed being single with no commitments or responsibilities, so our relationship faded out. It was fun while it lasted.

As 1993 progressed, my friends and acquaintances began fixing me up with different guys

A few of these "fix ups" never got further than a few phone calls. My attorney friend, **Stan**, wanted me to meet one of his colleagues. He had a very low nasal voice, which I found amusing. He introduced himself as **Herbie**, and told me that he was divorced but had been the best husband that anyone could ever have. He told me about his children and how lucky they were to have him. I don't know why, but that seemed like the longest fifteen minutes of my life. When he asked me about myself, I told him that I lived in Tarzana, causing him to let out a deep, nasal groan. "Oh," he said, "You live so far away from me. I live in The Borscht Belt."

He described the Borscht Belt as the very religious Jewish area of Los Angeles. He still wanted to meet me and suggested that we meet half way. I said that I could probably do that. Then he said that we would have to talk later because his children needed him, and after all, he was the best father that anyone could ever have.

Herbie called again about a week later. Sounding more nasal than usual, he told me that he had been in a car accident a few days earlier. Although he wasn't hurt, he was very shaken up and afraid to drive. He said that he would love to go out with me, but he wanted me to come and pick him up. I wished him well, suggested that he seek some therapy to over-come his fear of driving, and perhaps we could get together when he was emotionally stronger. Good Bye!

One Sunday in the spring, I was invited to a party at the home of my friends, Amy and Alan. While there, I met some lovely people. One woman named Ora, said that she had some men in mind to fix me up with, so she asked for my telephone number.

A nice looking man named **Jack** approached me and we

started talking. He and his family had been friends of Amy and Alan's for years. He was a second grade teacher, and since I had also taught school, we had a lot in common. He asked me for my telephone number.

I gave Jack my number. He called me the next day and asked me out to dinner the following Saturday night.

He picked me up at 7:00, and we drove into Malibu to his favorite dive, you should excuse the pun. That was our first major difference. The seating in the restaurant was very uncomfortable. The noise level was unbearable and the long tables and benches, family style, did not lend well to privacy, or even conversation, but as the evening went on, I discovered that his company wasn't much better. Jack spent the majority of the time whining about his financial difficulties and how his parents helped support him. A first date is not the best time to concentrate on negatives and to constantly whine. This wimpy man was definitely not my type.

While on the way home, Jack told me that we were going to be passing right by his apartment.

He very enthusiastically said, "Say! I just painted the ceiling of my apartment. How would you like to stop off and see it?"

I told him that I needed to get home (badly) and perhaps he could take me to see his ceiling another time.

Jack was visibly disappointed when I declined his lovely invitation.

When we arrived back at my place, I thanked Jack for a pleasant evening, and before I knew it, he kissed me right on the mouth with his tongue jutting half way down my throat! I slammed my mouth shut, got out of the car and ran upstairs and washed my mouth out with mouthwash! What a night.

About a week later, Ora called me and told me that she had given my number to a very nice Israeli contractor who had done some work for her husband. Later that evening, **Avi** called. He had a thick accent and it took me time to adjust to it. He seemed nice, so I accepted a dinner date for the following Thursday night.

Thursday night, 7:30 sharp, my phone rang. Avi was at the security gate. I buzzed him in, and told him to meet me by my garage. I ran outside to meet him, and to my surprise, he pulled up in a beat up pick-up truck. He stopped, rolled the window down, and told me to open the door and jump in. As I jumped in the truck, I looked up at my dining room window. All three of my boys were laughing hysterically while pointing to me in the old pick-up truck. I smiled at them and waved.

When Avi greeted me, I immediately smelled whiskey and cigarettes on his breath. What an instant turn off.

He was in the mood for Chinese food, so I suggested a good place nearby. As we pulled up to the restaurant, I had forgotten that there was valet parking. What a sight we were, pulling up to the valet in the old truck!

We were seated at a lovely table and while we waited for our food, Avi talked about his nasty divorce and revealed that I was his first post-divorce date.

As I listened, I couldn't help but fixate on his mouth. He had about the worst case of gingivitis that I had ever seen.

Avi told me that he couldn't understand why his wife divorced him. It's true that he smacked her around a bit, but she deserved it. Oh boy!

Dinner wasn't over soon enough. I told Avi that I had to get home right away to my children. Children sure came in handy when excuses were needed!

When we pulled up at my townhouse, he asked if he could call me again. I told him that perhaps he needed more time to deal with the emotions of his divorce. I then extended my hand for a friendly handshake, jumped out of the truck, and ran inside.

Ora called the next day and anxiously wanted to know how the date went with Avi. I began by telling her how much I appreciated her efforts, but although Avi was a nice man, he wasn't for me. Ora was so sweet. She said that she was sorry and proceeded to tell me about another man that she wanted me to meet. What did I have to lose? I told her to go ahead and give him my number.

The next day, he called. His name was **Monty** and he was also newly divorced and living in Pasadena. He was also Israeli, but was much easier to understand. He asked me out for the following Friday night. When he arrived, he drove a jeep, and the boys seemed rather disappointed. They were all set for another big laugh.

Monty was a very good-looking man with blond hair. He was bright and warm. He took me out for Mexican food and then we went to a French restaurant for coffee and dessert. He was still quite raw since his divorce and he was in the midst of fighting for full custody of his two young boys. Monty's great passion was going sky diving every weekend. He had been a sky-diver in the Israeli army at one time, and kept up the hobby. He was very enthusiastic about getting me to try it. No way, no way, no way!

When we returned to my townhouse, Monty was in a very loving, affectionate mood. A little too much for me. I told him so, and he was a real gentleman. He then left after asking me out for the following Monday night.

I still saw Jeff about once every weekend. The relationship was much less frustrating for me while I had these other experiences going on in my life. Even if the dates were less than ideal, it was quite refreshing to know that other men were attracted to me.

The following Monday night, Marta arrived to babysit, as usual. I was ready, anxiously awaiting Monty's arrival. At the exact time that he was supposed to pick me up, he called. He sounded quite upset. He told me that he had his children for the day, and his ex-wife never arrived to pick them up. I was disappointed, but sympathized with him. I was really looking forward to our date. He told me to wait a little longer and maybe she would come to get them. Forty minutes later he called. The ex-wife finally arrived and took the children. Monty then told me that he was exhausted and he asked me to drive out to his place in Pasadena. I didn't want to make the same mistake that I made with Jeff. I suggested that he come to me. He seemed quite put out, and we said goodbye. He never called again.

I felt badly because I liked Monty. I called Ora and told her what had happened, and she told me that she would talk to him and get back to me. A few days later, she called. She had finally spoken to Monty, and evidently he was having some real problems with the ex-wife and decided not to get involved with anyone else until he had his life straightened out.

Ora, still not giving up on me, told me that she knew of another man. This man's name was **Dave** and she had also briefly met him through her husband's work. Although she didn't really know him, she said that he was really handsome and that we would make an outstanding looking couple. He evidently looked like Richard Gere. I thanked her for the compliment and told her once again that it would be okay to give him my number.

A few days later, around 9:00 P.M., Dave called. "Hello, Kathy, dis is Dave. Ora gave me dis number to call you. Where do you live? I am not familiar with dis particular area code."

I tried to maintain my composure while I answered him. I couldn't believe the way he spoke. I told him where I lived and I asked him where he was living.

"I been living in a room at my good friend's house out at da base of da San Gabriel Mountains. Oh, can you hold on for a minute?"

He then proceeded to talk to some children who had obviously entered the room. "Get outa here kids. I'm on a very important call. Leave da room!"

I heard one of the children answer him by saying, "You're in big trouble Dave, because Dad says you aren't allowed to use the phone!"

After a few more minutes on hold, Dave finally came back on the line. "Ya see, I don't got any money now. I went bankrupt a few years ago, and I just got outa da County Hospital. I been sick, but no one knows what da problem is. Da doctors can't do all the tests on me dat they'd like to do 'cause I don't got no insurance."

Maybe this guy was good looking, but that's about all he had going for him. He then said, Oh Kathy, I gotta go. It's almost 10:00, and I gotta meet da buddies at da bowling alley."

I told him that it seemed really late to start bowling. Dave then said, "At dis bowling alley dat I go to, after 10:00 P.M. you can bowl a game for 75 cents! Dat's about all I can afford."

We wrapped up this stimulating conversation, and when Dave suggested that it would be nice to get together, I told him that we really lived much too far apart. He said, "Ah, dat's too bad."

Just then the children and their dad came into the room and screamed at Dave to get off of the phone.

I couldn't wait for Ora's next pick.

Bettylou called me a few days later and after I shared my

newest experiences with her, we both had a good laugh. Then she told me that a mutual friend of ours, Jerry Hanson, had asked Bettylou if she thought that it was okay to call me and ask me out. This was a rather touchy situation because Jerry and his wife, Sylvia, had recently split up. I had been friends with both of them.

Jerry called me that night and he asked me to go with him to the The Whiskey to see a punk band that he liked. I agreed to go; however, I was rather leery about going to The Whiskey, because it mostly catered to teenagers, and I wasn't much into punk music.

Jerry picked me up for our date, and as we drove to the Sunset Strip, we got reacquainted, since I hadn't really seen him or his wife since their separation. After hearing the sad details of their separation, I could tell that Jerry was in a mid life crisis, trying to regain his teenage years again.

We had dinner on the Sunset Strip, and then we drove to the Whiskey. As we stood in line to enter, I felt really uncomfortable. We were clearly the oldest couple there, although Jerry was like a teenager again. He was so excited to hear this group, he could hardly contain himself. Finally the doors opened and we were ushered into the club. We were the only couple that wasn't required to show proof of age at the door. My feet were very tired after standing in line for so long. I couldn't wait to be seated. To my dismay, this club was standing room only. To make things worse, they packed us in like sardines. Jerry looked very happy, obviously used to this set up.

The group came on the stage, and the crowd got so excited, that we were almost knocked over and stomped on. The music began, and the kids around me started jumping and head bashing. The musical group was certainly not my style. Neither was this crowd. I couldn't believe Jerry. He was really into the music. For a moment I thought that he was going to start head bashing. I was really scared that we were going to get hurt. The crowd around us was becoming more and more hyper. I told Jerry that I just couldn't stay there. He then led me upstairs where it wasn't quite as wild, but just as loud.

By the time it ended, I was miserable, but Jerry was really charged up and elated. This was one of the best concerts he had been to in a long time. Oh boy!

We then walked back to Jerry's car. He asked me if I would like to hear another punk band playing down the street. When I declined the offer, he proceeded to drive like a maniac all the way home. I told him to please slow down. I was really afraid for my life. When we arrived at my house, I thanked God that we actually made it home without getting into an accident.

Jerry thanked me for joining him and asked if I was up to going to another concert with him the following week. I declined once again, telling him that I was quite busy for the next few weeks (months, and years).

My friends, Ronna and Barry, called. They wanted to fix me up with a good friend of theirs named Joel. Joel was quite a bit older than I, having just turned fifty-five, but they convinced me that he was quite youthful for his age.

Joel called a few days later, and after an enjoyable conversation, we made plans to go for dinner later that week. Joel was a very nice man and I enjoyed our dinner date together. We continued to date for a few weeks. He was very thoughtful and nice to my boys, even bringing them gifts when he went out of town. All seemed to be going well until one evening when he proceeded to tell me that he was kind of into S & M. (sadomasochism). He said that he belonged to an organization of people who also were into this thing. He enthusiastically showed me a current newsletter published by the organization. I was practically speechless. He then told me that the next "get together" was in a couple of weeks and he wanted me to go with him. When I started to decline his offer, Joel told me that I would be surprised to see who the people were. He said that I could very well see my own doctor or dentist there. I didn't want to see them there! Sensing my apprehensive look, Joel told me that I had nothing to worry about. Nobody would force me to participate. It would be okay to just watch.

This was unbelievable. I told Joel that I was in no way interested in this type of activity. When he looked disappointed, I apologized, but reiterated that I was not interested in going with him.

That was the end of my brief relationship with Joel. When I told Ronna about this latest discovery about Joel, she was shocked. She and Barry had no idea that Joel was into that kind of activity.

It sure wasn't easy being single again, especially at my age. Many of the men were either badly divorced or had commitment problems. Or the chemistry just wasn't there. This dating scene was rather discouraging, but I wasn't giving up. I still hoped to find a soul mate in life, and this would take patience and time.

Gail, one of the girls in Gary's widow/widowers support group became one of my very closest friends. I met her at the widow/widower social, where I met Gary. She too, was actively dating and having about as much luck as I. She was in a relationship with a man that was in many ways similar to Jeff. A common bond was solidified by our daily commiseration over these men. Gail and I kept our spirits up with our frequent conversations and whenever we didn't have dates on the weekend, we would go out together. We enjoyed each other's company more than we enjoyed most of our dates. We did a lot of laughing and crying together. This is what kept us afloat.

The summer of 1993 arrived, and with it continual frustration with Jeff. While dating other men, I wasn't so focused on the negativity of the relationship. I was getting closer to calling it quits with him. It took time to build up the courage to say goodbye, and release the fear of possibly being alone again. At the time I just didn't understand that I was alone even when we were together.

Around the beginning of July, I received a phone call from my old boyfriend, **Ken Weston**. I attended my high school prom with him, and ended up going to the same university as he. We broke up in college, but Ken always remained in touch with me. He was very upset when I married Sandy, as he always thought that we would get back together. After Ken graduated from college he went on to law school, and then on to a position in a prestigious firm. After breaking up, we lost contact for quite a while, and it wasn't until I was engaged to be married that he called me again and wanted to know if we could give it another try. The timing was all wrong. I was getting married to Sandy two days later. Ken tried to talk me out of it, and when he saw that it was useless, he vowed that he would always keep in touch no matter where he was. He was true to his word.

Ken ended up marrying a girl he had met back east. He

never sounded really thrilled about her, but he said that she took good care of him. I was so proud of his achievements. He did not come from a wealthy family and had to work his way through school. He attributed part of his success in law to my father, who inspired him to excel.

When Sandy died, he called periodically to see how I was doing. He told me that he really wanted to see me, but his wife would just not permit it, even a platonic lunch. She evidently was extremely jealous of me, knowing of our past relationship and how he felt about me.

So that summer, Ken called me. This phone call was different from the others because he told me that he was very unhappily married. His wife and children were back east visiting his wife's family and he was home alone for two weeks. He desperately wanted to see me. I agreed to see him, although I was clear that we would have to remain platonic as long as he was married. That was difficult to say because I was very vulnerable and, truthfully, I always cared about him.

Ken drove out to the valley to pick me up for the day. When I saw him, it was as if time had stood still for twenty some years. He looked absolutely wonderful. We had a wonderful day together. We went to Laguna Beach and walked and talked, and then went for drinks at the Ritz Carlton Hotel. Afterwards, Ken took me to his home. He was very excited to show me where he lived. Not surprising, his house was beautiful. He turned me towards him and held me close and whispered into my ear, "See what you could have had if you had married me."

I was speechless. It was true. I felt as if I had really blown things. We probably could have been very happy together.

When we returned to the valley, we stopped for dinner at a restaurant that we always used to go to when we were teenagers. While we were eating our burgers and talking and laughing, all of a sudden Ken stopped talking, looked at me, and said, "I love you."

I said, "What did you say?"

He said, "Kathy, I love you and I have never stopped loving you in all the years that we have known one another."

I started to cry. It felt so good to hear that he really cared about me. I also had never stopped loving him.

Seeing Ken now, I truly questioned the choices I had made. I was now free, but he was very married. I wanted to know his intentions. I didn't want to be hurt.

Knowing how I felt, Ken said that the last thing he wanted was to hurt me. He told me that he had been in therapy for quite a while, and my name kept coming up. He was so torn. He wanted a life with me, yet he was terrified of what his wife could take from him if he divorced her. He worked so hard to get everything that he had, and he wasn't about to lose any of it in divorce.

Although we saw each other a few more times, I knew that it could never go any further. I just enjoyed the time we had together. This was a real ego boost for me! I have had very little contact with him since my remarriage.

Around the same time that summer, Bettylou and Barry told me that they had someone for me to meet. He was a colleague of Barry's living in Chicago. **Ed** was the host of an all night radio show. He was in L.A. interviewing for a television position on MTV. Bettylou said that I would enjoy him, although because of the gypsy life of a radio personality, she would not consider him as a long-term prospect. He sounded like fun, so I agreed to go over to Bettylou's house on a Friday night for drinks, and then out to dinner with Bettylou, Barry, and Ed.

When I arrived at their house, I was pleasantly surprised. Ed was everything that my friends said about him, and more. He was charming, extremely intelligent, warm, vivacious, and good looking! I was very impressed with him, and felt quite complimented when he expressed his positive feelings for me.

The four of us had a fabulous dinner at Barry and Bettylou's favorite restaurant, and then we returned to their house and sat outdoors in candlelight, talking for hours. When it was time for me to go, Ed walked me out to my car, kissed me, and asked me to spend the rest of the weekend with him and Bettylou and Barry. Then he told me that he wanted to take me out to dinner before his flight back to Chicago early the next week.

The weekend was wonderful. Ed made me feel so good. Between Ed and Ken, I said to myself, "Jeff who?" In fact, it felt good telling Jeff that I was busy all weekend. But being my foolish self, I agreed to see him during the week.

Before Ed left, he took me out to a romantic dinner down

at Paradise Cove in Malibu. We had such a wonderful time. I would miss his vibrant personality and passion for life. He was one of the most exciting men that I had ever been with. He will always hold a very dear place in my heart.

Summer was passing fast, and before I knew it, it was mid August and soccer season was beginning. All three of the boys would be playing again. Adam's coach was Morrie, who had coached him with Sandy a few years earlier, and Tom Edwin was the assistant coach.

Tom was a darling man who had also been Adam's assistant coach the season before. He was a successful producer and recently divorced. One day soon after the season began, I was sitting in my usual spot watching the practice. He came up behind me, wrapped his arms around me, and gave me a big hug. Shocked, I turned around to see who this was. I was really happy to see that it was Tom.

He sat down beside me and asked, "Kathy, how are you doing?"

I said, "I'm doing fine."

"I'm divorced now."

I said, "I'm so sorry to hear this."

"Oh, don't be sorry," he responded. "I'm very relieved that it is finally over. I think that you are so lovely and I have been attracted to you ever since I met you a year ago. But because I wasn't divorced yet, I didn't want to start anything with you. Are you in a relationship with anyone right now?"

I told him briefly about my ridiculous relationship with Jeff.

He said, "Oh Kathy, you poor thing. You are too beautiful of a person to be treated that way. I would love to take you out and treat you like you deserve to be treated."

I was thrilled to hear this and very excited to go out with him. We planned to go out the following Saturday night. He said that he wanted to get together sooner, but he had to go out of town to shoot a commercial.

I could hardly wait for our date. While Tom was away, he called me several times, and even though it was long distance, we talked for over two hours. He would tell me about the circumstances of his divorce, and I told him what I went through when

Sandy died. We seemed to be good for each other.

Finally Saturday arrived. When he came to pick me up, he was so warm and loving with the boys. They all thought that he was terrific.

We drove to Universal City to the City Walk to have dinner and go to the movies. While we were driving there he confided that I was his first date since his divorce. He said that it felt a little strange, but good. He had been married for twenty years.

We had dinner, walked around holding hands, and then we went into the movies. Half way into the movie, Tom was paged. He excused himself and went out to make a call to his home. He came back about ten minutes later visibly upset. I asked him what was wrong. He told me that his five-year-old son, who was at his house this weekend, was having a lot of emotional problems because of the divorce. He was crying and wanted his daddy. I understood, and although I hated our evening to end, I told him that he probably should get home. He agreed, and he drove me home. He apologized, told me that he'd see me at the next practice, and he left.

I didn't see Tom at practice that week because he was out of town. The following Saturday, I saw him at the soccer games. He ran over to me, gave me a big hug and kiss, and took me and my boys, with his boys to lunch at a nearby diner. I asked him how his children were doing, and he said that it was going to take time. They were all in therapy.

Whenever I went to practice, Tom was always waiting for me with open arms, but because of the emotional circumstances of his family, we never seemed to get it together.

One Sunday afternoon, Tom invited us to his place. His own children were not there that day. He seemed depressed and a little distant. I knew that he was missing his children.

After that day, Tom and I never got together again. On one occasion, after a soccer game, he invited the boys to go with him to a hockey game. The boys were excited. He told me that he would call me later with the details. He never did. The boys were devastated. I explained to them that Tom was going through a difficult time in his life, and although he meant well, we couldn't rely on him.

The end of Jeff

I was again down to seeing Jeff on the weekends. As my birthday approached, Jeff talked about taking me for dinner. The Wednesday before my Saturday birthday, Jeff called me. He said, "Kathy, I know that you are probably expecting me to take you for dinner on your birthday."

I responded, "Yes, you had implied that a while ago."

"Well, something has come up and I won't be able to take you. A very important friend in my community is having a birthday party for his wife, and I really have to go."

That creep. He didn't even have the decency to include me. This sounded very fishy. He then went on to say that he couldn't take me out the following Saturday night because he needed to spend more time with his children.

I was understandably outraged. My girlfriends told me to dump him, as they had told me many times before. I was finally becoming strong enough emotionally to get rid of him and not accept any more of his abuse.

Jeff did not call that week. I was furious and had no desire to speak to him either. I was waiting for an apology from him. It never came.

The Saturday night following my birthday, Gail and I were having dinner together. She wanted to help me decide to erase him from my life. When I told her that Jeff said that he was going to spend this Saturday night with his children, Gail suggested that we call him. I really didn't want to know the truth. She told me that I better face up to it.

I agreed to the phone call. Gail would call, and if Jeff answered, she would hang up. If one of the children answered, she would ask to speak to their father. I felt like we were teenagers placing a prank call, but we were both really curious.

At about 8:00 P.M., I dialed Jeff's number from a pay phone and then handed the receiver to Gail. The line rang a couple of times, and then Gail said, "Hi! Is your dad home?" Then a few seconds passed and Gail said, "Oh, this is a friend of your dad's, but I'll call back when he's home. By the way, do you know what time he'll be home?"

I couldn't believe Gail was doing this. I was dying.

"Okay." Gail responded into the receiver, "There's no

message."

"Well?" I asked Gail.

"You were right. He's not home with his children and they don't know when to expect him. You've been had." Gail replied honestly.

I was hurt, but not surprised. I had long known that I didn't deserve this type of rejection. If he didn't want to see me anymore, he could have been a man about it and confronted me. But then again, wasn't I expecting too much from an insensitive, selfish man?

I never heard from Jeff again. To have adequate closure, I wrote him a short, simple note on a piece of stationery with my letterhead on it. The note simply said:

> I am so disappointed in you as a person.
> You have hurt me so deeply.
> You could have had the decency to say goodbye.

I didn't sign it. I just addressed it and sent it. I never heard another word from him again.

Car trouble

To add to my frustrations, the car that my parents had given me after Sandy died, was dying as well. On numerous occasions I was stranded with the boys because the car wouldn't start. No one was able to diagnose this problem because it was intermittent. I was in constant fear of being stranded in the dangerous neighborhoods associated with my apartment management job, and not knowing if I would have reliable transportation for my children. It was time to get a new car.

I was able to purchase a new Honda LX Accord with some of the leftover life insurance. Getting my beautiful new car made me so happy. It was paid for in full, eliminating the nightmare of large car payments that I had dealt with in my marriage.

Dating continues

November came, and with it new experiences. One of the mothers from Jordan's class fixed me up with her financial planner. **Sam** had been married once briefly and had no children. He was a very handsome and sweet guy, and we seemed to have a lot in common.

At the end of our first date, Sam invited me to go out to dinner with him and two other couples. He said that he wanted his friends to meet me. I was delighted to go. This invitation was a breath of fresh air for me, so different from my negative relationship with Jeff, who wouldn't introduce me to anybody.

Sam's friends were very warm and open. Sam made me feel good and seemed proud to have me with him.

We saw each other the following weekend. The weekend after that, he invited me to go down to San Pedro with him for the day. He grew up there, and still had some friends that lived in the area. He wanted to visit his friends before the holidays and introduce them to me. He also was eager to show me where he had lived and gone to school. We had a great time.

Sam asked if I would like to take a few days off at Christmas and go up the coast to Monterey with him. That sounded great. I then invited him to spend Christmas with us, at my brother, Rick's house. My parents would be there as well. He was delighted to join us.

Christmas came, and Sam drove out to Rick's with us. My whole family enjoyed his company. He had a great sense of humor and was a lot of fun. He bought the boys an air hockey table, which he assembled with them when we returned home. He bought me a gorgeous sweater. Things seemed to be going well.

Toward the end of the Christmas season, Sam started complaining that his throat hurt and he felt like he was coming down with something. Since we were to leave for Monterey in a couple of days, I suggested that he see a doctor. He told me that he did not have any medical insurance and he didn't want to spend the money to see a doctor. Here he was a financial planner with no physician and no medical insurance.

Bettylou and Ronna each offered to take the boys while I was out of town.

When we were all set to go, Sam asked if we could take my car. I wasn't very happy about this request because my car was practically brand new and I didn't want to drive it so hard at first. He told me that the lease was almost up on his Chevy Blazer, and he did not want to put unnecessary mileage on it.

I'm sure that he figured that I might back out and that was why he waited until the last minute when all the plans were made. This didn't feel good. A little red flag went up.

We ended up taking my car. We dropped the children off and began our drive up the coast. Things didn't feel right to me. Sam was very quiet, and when I asked him what was wrong, he told me that he didn't feel well. I suggested that perhaps this wasn't the best time for him to travel. He snapped at me saying that he never went anywhere anymore, and he needed a vacation. We drove the rest of the way in silence.

Monterey was beautiful, but the company was disappointing. Sam was a major drag. We spent a great deal of time in pharmacies picking out "economical" over-the-counter medications for him. He spent most of the vacation time whining about his throat. I knew that we shouldn't have gone.

I was glad when we arrived back home. I had invited him to a New Year's party at Ronna and Barry's house, and hoped that he would feel better by then.

He never did see a doctor, and was too sick to be with me on New Year's Eve. He told me that he had to go to his office and work, and that was about all that he could handle. Sam did not feel well enough to come to the New Year's Day party with me either. I had a great time anyway, celebrating the beginning of 1994 with my friends. It was rather refreshing not hearing anyone whine about his health.

Sam slowly recovered from his virus. I didn't see much of him because he claimed that he needed to devote all of his time to catch up on things at work. He did suggest that since he was a financial planner that perhaps I should consider letting him handle my money. We met at his office, and he presented a financial plan. I was not impressed and didn't think that it would be a good idea to get him involved in my personal affairs.

Sam was visibly disappointed with my decision, and I was becoming more and more disillusioned with him and knew that it was time to move on.

The earthquake

As if life wasn't complicated enough, we were awakened by the terrifying mid-January earthquake. It was a little after 4:00

in the morning, and suddenly our townhouse started shaking violently, causing everything to fall and break around us. Things were falling off of the shelves, furniture was falling over, and I could hear the constant breaking of glass, along with the crashing down of televisions, stereo equipment, pictures, crystal, and almost everything else. The boys were screaming hysterically, and I jumped out of bed while the shaking was still going on, attempting to make it to the boys' room. I crawled through broken glass strewn all over the hallway, among remnants of what used to be family pictures hung on my wall.

It seemed like an eternity before I got to the boys' room. Grabbing each of them out of bed and placing them in their doorway for safety, I crawled through the debris of what used to be on their shelves, to get to their closet for their shoes. It was difficult to see, because it was still dark outside, and there was no power. After feeling around in the dark and locating their shoes, we rushed downstairs. Jamie had fallen asleep on the couch downstairs, and he was hysterically crying and calling for me. I told him to run to the guest bathroom doorway and wait for me. When he was running to the doorway, the VCR flew off the top of the large screen TV and hit him in the head, practically knocking him out. I just couldn't believe this was happening. I really thought that this was "the big one," and that we were all going to die. I wasn't giving up though. Finally, the shaking stopped, temporarily. The boys and I were able to make it downstairs and go to Jamie. Then we grabbed coats in the closet next to the front door, and ran outside, out of the reach of electrical wires and falling glass.

I was relieved to join all of our neighbors outside. They were all so good to us, knowing that I was alone with the boys. One of the neighbors from the other side of our townhouse ran over to me and told me that water was gushing out of my garage. A group of men living across the alley ran over and manually opened my garage where we discovered that my water heater had broken from the wall and burst open, flooding the entire area. Everything that had been on the shelves, had fallen on to my new car, denting in the hood. I carefully pulled the car out. Everyone else was doing the same, just in case the garages would collapse and trap our vehicles. We could feel after-shocks every few minutes, some very strong.

Finally, daybreak came. We all cautiously entered our units to inspect the damages. It looked like a bomb blast. Everything had fallen to the ground and most things were broken. My crystal was shattered, all of my kitchen appliances were destroyed, dishes and glasses were all broken, and liquor bottles had flown out of the top cabinet and crashed in tiny, sticky pieces all over the floor.

Upstairs, all of our bedroom furniture had fallen over, and clothing was strewn all over the floor. Everything that had once been up, was now down. One of the toilets even broke loose from the floor of the bathroom.

I quickly gathered clothing and toiletries and packed them up. It would be quite a while before we could live here again. I left before more aftershocks could place me in additional danger.

I tried to reach my parents, but because of the power outage over much of Los Angeles, my phone didn't work. Finally one of my neighbors let me use his cellular phone. My parents were frantic because they couldn't reach us. They said that they were okay, and luckily they did not have the devastation that we had. They lived in the mountains and it appeared to be safer. We would later find out that our townhouse was practically at the epicenter.

The boys and I went to my parents' house to stay with them. They still had power and running water. We had nothing at the townhouse.

Before we left, I called my friends to make sure they were okay, and then I called Sam to see how he was. He was badly shaken up, and seemed to have quite a bit of damage, although not as much damage as I had. I told him that if he wanted to talk, he could reach me at my parents' house. I didn't hear from him.

We stayed with my parents for a week. During the day, I returned to the townhouse to clean up the horrible mess. My mother came with me the first day, and when she saw the debris, she said that she thought that it was a miracle that we were still alive!

I didn't own the townhouse, but almost everything I owned had to be replaced. I received some government disaster relief money to help me replace some necessary items. My sister-in-law,

Sheila, also sent us some money to help us. That was so kind and generous of her, and very unexpected.

When we returned to live in the townhouse, the children and I were still very nervous and apprehensive. For about a week we slept in sweat suits, with flashlights next to us, near the front door, like many people. It would take a while to recover from the trauma.

Slowly, we became more used to the diminishing after-shocks, and life began to get back to normal. It would be over a year before all the necessary repairs would be completed in and around our townhouse.

During the tumult following the earthquake, I once again began to think about Sandy in his grave. Did the earthquake shake his coffin? Was he now in a different position? Was he still clutching our photos and the letters? I had such morbid thoughts. It's interesting that the boys never thought of this morbidity. As time passed, the boys and I began to think of Sandy's remains less frequently and focused more on the living memories that we had of him.

In late January, Sam called. He was very friendly and told me that he was sorry for not calling for a while, but work was really hectic. He wanted to know if he could come over to my place to watch the Super Bowl on my large screen TV. I told him that it would be okay, since the boys would be watching it anyway.

When he left that evening, he apologized for not being more attentive, and once again, he blamed it on his work and his mental state following the earthquake. I accepted his apology, and wished him well.

Sam and I sort of fizzled out. We met a couple of times for coffee during the day when he was between appointments in the valley, but that was it. A couple of months later, he called and told me that his dad had just passed away. He was very broken up. I offered my condolences and wished him well. That was the last time I heard from him. Another guy, another relationship.

Do I need a man?

The dating scene was becoming very disillusioning and I came to the conclusion that I really didn't need a man to survive.

If I continued to meet men like these, maybe I was better off alone. It was a relief to be unattached for a while. I was finally developing the security and emotional stability that I had lacked all of my adult life. I would never let any man abuse me ever again. This emotional growth felt wonderful. I felt good about myself, and I vowed that if I ever remarried, it would be to a man who respected and appreciated me.

Being a single parent was difficult. But as disillusioned as I was, I am optimistic by nature. Raising three active, strong-willed boys by myself presented an exhausting challenge. It was difficult to be a consistently strong mother. I felt sorry for the boys, losing their father at such a young age. This sorrow softened me and I wasn't the firm and consistent disciplinarian that I should have been. I was also emotionally drained, so it was very easy for the boys to manipulate me to get what they wanted. They knew how vulnerable I was and very often took advantage. Any man I might marry would be taking on a big responsibility handling these boys. I might not have needed a man in order to survive, but I knew that the boys needed a good, strong father figure in their lives. Being a mom, this was something that I was not able to give them.

I reminded my optimistic self that the situation that I was in now did not have to be permanent. Improvements were in reach.

The amazing psychic

One Wednesday night in late February, The Widow Pam called and asked me if I was available on Saturday night. I said yes, and asked her what she had in mind. She and a few of the other widows from our group were going to hear a prominent psychic speak at a nearby hotel. She wanted to know if I would like to join them. I was slightly apprehensive, but agreed to go.

The Widow Pam picked me up and we drove together to the hotel. We were the last two people to be let in without reservations.

The room was brightly lit, the same as any other room designed for business seminars. Our other widow friends were already there and seated in the front of the room. We sat near the back of the room where we would be able to see the psychic, but the psychic would not be able to see us. I was still a little spooked by the whole idea of the evening, so I was very content with this seating arrangement.

The psychic entered and took his place up in the front. He introduced himself as James Van Praagh. He seemed like any ordinary person, but he displayed a terrific personality. I was very pleasantly surprised. He put us at ease as soon as he began to speak.

Mr. Van Praagh began by telling us all about himself and how he discovered his psychic abilities. He was fascinating. He conducted a relaxation exercise, and then he said that he was ready to begin.

He explained that he had a spiritual guide who helped him contact those who had passed over. The place where we all go when we pass over is peaceful and beautiful, with the colors more vibrant than here, and the sounds clearer. When one passes over, they still maintain a job or profession, but it is usually on a higher level. He explained that if a man had been a construction worker when he was living, then when he passed over, he would perhaps be an architect. He went on to say that spirits who have moved on and passed over, can still return to visit us if they are strongly thought about or summoned. There wasn't enough time for all the spirits to come to us tonight, and only the strongest spirits would be able to communicate.

I didn't know what to think about all of this. It was really hard to believe all of the things that he talked about, yet it was all very interesting.

Mr. Van Praagh became very quiet, and the room went silent. After a few minutes, he said, "Someone is here who has 'passed over.' It's a boy, a young child. Has anyone in this room lost a young boy?"

After about thirty seconds, a woman sitting in the fourth row from the front, slowly and timidly raised her hand.

Mr. Van Praagh walked over to her and said, "Momma, Poppa, I'm okay. I'm happy here where you buried me." He then said to the woman, "Your son is buried far away from here. In...it's coming to me...it's a place that starts with an E..."

The woman was crying. She said that her son was buried in Eaglerock.

He then said to the woman, "He tells me that you were not happy with his burial location. He wants you to know that it's okay. He's buried in his baseball uniform and cap, and he's happy."

The woman was crying harder than ever. She said that she and her family fought about the location of her son's burial and he was buried in a place that did not meet with her approval. She said that she didn't feel that he would be happy there. "Yes," the poor woman said, "my little boy was buried in his baseball uniform and cap." Then she promptly got up, still crying, and ran out of the room.

I couldn't believe this. It appeared to be real. As I sat there, I could hear the people around me gasping. They were as shocked as I.

Then, after a few moments of silence, Mr. Van Praagh asked which of us had eaten a huge chocolate cookie before coming here tonight. There was a rather long silence and he asked again. "Okay, which one of you ate this huge cookie?"

A rather plump woman sitting in the fifth row from the front reluctantly raised her hand. Mr. Van Praagh walked over to her and asked her who had "passed over" whose name was Rose?"

She timidly looked up at him and said that Rose was her grandmother who had died recently.

He then said, "Rose says that you've been doing so well on that new diet, so why did you eat that big cookie?"

We all started to laugh, again in utter disbelief that this was all really happening. By the way, the woman was there alone, so no one could have known that she had eaten that cookie, or that she had a grandmother named Rose.

As the evening went on, Mr. Van Praagh contacted more spirits. I was having a fabulous time. He returned after a short intermission, and the evening continued. I wasn't ready for what was about to happen.

Mr. Van Praagh, still standing in the front of the room said, "There's someone here who has 'passed over.' He's having a great deal of difficulty breathing. It's his heart, no...it's his lungs. It's awful. He's got...lung cancer. Who in this room has lost someone from lung cancer?"

I was in shock. Pam elbowed my arm to encourage me to overcome my unaccustomed shyness. Slowly I raised my hand. I could hear the people stirring around me.

Mr. Van Praagh walked over to where he could see me. "He was your husband. He's, he's very pissed off! Wow, he's a tough man. He's a good man, but a tough man. He's pissed off because he doesn't like the color he turned in the hospital."

I couldn't believe this. It's true. Because Sandy's liver was filled with cancer, he was terribly jaundiced. Being a very vain person, if he had been alert, he would have been quite alarmed and upset with his color.

Mr. Van Praagh continued. "The three children, boys...tell them I miss them. Tell them that I spend a lot of time in the top bunk."

Oh my god, the boys have bunk beds and Adam, whose appearance is identical to his father, sleeps in the top bunk!

"I'm getting something about a wallet. He's upset about a wallet. Do you have his wallet?"

I told him that I did have his wallet. Then it dawned on me that just recently the Louis Vuitton wallet that he had bought me years ago needed to be replaced. I didn't want to spend a lot of money on it, so I purchased an inexpensive wallet. Because it was cheap, it broke practically immediately, and had to be exchanged. Then the new one broke. I knew that if Sandy had been alive, he wouldn't have approved of a cheap wallet. He always said that you get what you pay for. I was convinced that this was a signal from Sandy that he disapproved of my wallet selection.

Mr. Van Praagh then went on to say, "Your husband is having great difficulty communicating. Some spirits come through strong and vital and colorful. Your husband is a hazy gray. Oh, he says that you have just received money from someone whose name starts with an 'S'. It's...Sherry, no, Shawna, no...Sheila."

Oh God! Sheila had given me money after the earthquake. No one knew about this. There was no way that he could have known! I started to silently cry. So did everyone around me.

Mr. Van Praagh went on. "Tell the boys I love them." Then he walked closer to me and said, "Your husband is very concerned about your headaches." Everyone gasped around me. I just nodded my head and silently wept. "Your husband says that maybe you should have your blood checked. Maybe there is something that will show up in your blood that is causing your headaches."

It was true. I had been suffering from migraine headaches for years. Sandy had felt very badly about my suffering and was always hopeful that I would find a remedy.

After about thirty seconds, he said, "He says that you will be asked by a man to go away on a trip. Go. Enjoy. Be happy. I love you. I love you."

Then it was over. I was still crying and shaking. People around me were offering comfort. How did he know these things? There were other things that he said that I can't recall, but everything he said was true. Some things that he said could be considered general, but most were specific. He had not been fed information, nor had I discussed anything before the evening began or at intermission.

None of my other widow friends were contacted. Afterwards, I felt a calm that stayed with me for quite a while. I felt at peace and that finally I had some closure.

Gary and I get a little closer

In mid-March, our Widow/Widowers Support Group had one of their social functions at a French restaurant in the valley. As usual, I was thrilled to see Gary there, and, as usual, we sat together.

I reiterated to Gary how disillusioned I was with the past men in my life. I asked him why they were such jerks. He said that I just hadn't met the right guy yet, but it would happen. He told me to be patient. I asked him how his relationship was going. He said that it had its ups and downs and he wasn't totally thrilled with the way things were developing. I told him not to settle for anyone who might not make him happy. He deserved so much. I suggested that maybe she wasn't the right one for him since there were already problems. I tried to be careful about my words because I didn't want to push him in any direction. He didn't respond.

Another widower named **Chad**, sat across from us. He was nice looking, very gentle, sensitive, and friendly. His wife had been killed in a car accident five years earlier, when their first child was only a few weeks old, and he was raising his son by himself.

I had a very nice conversation with Chad, and suggested that we get together sometime. He said that would be great, and he would give me a call.

A few weeks later, I still hadn't heard from Chad. I was somewhat interested in him. I called Gary and told him the situation and asked him if he thought I was being too pushy if I called Chad. Gary said to go ahead and call him. He told me that if he were really interested in me, Chad would be happy to hear from me. He felt that Chad was probably too shy to make the first call.

So, I called Chad. He wasn't home, so I left a detailed and warm message on his answering machine. A couple of hours later, he called me back. He told me that he was very happy to hear from me, and we made plans to go out for dinner that weekend. I was really happy, and looked forward to our date.

I called Gary and thanked him for his advice. He asked me what night I was going out with Chad. I told him, Friday night. He then asked me if I would like to go out to dinner and to a movie with him on Saturday night, just as friends, of course. I asked him what was going on with his relationship. He told me that the two of them were taking a hiatus from one another. They were having some problems, and Gary needed time to think.

I was looking forward to my weekend.

Chad and I had a great time and we arranged to get together the following Saturday night. Chad confessed to me that the only thing that he could think of while we were at the Widow/Widower social event, was how he wanted to drag me out to the parking lot and make wild and passionate love. I got such a kick out of this statement because Chad was such a reserved and quiet man!

Gary and I went to dinner, as planned, and while we were waiting for the movie, we browsed in a nearby bookstore. He was looking in the "relationship" section, while I looked in the "dating" section. After he purchased a book on how to make a relationship work, we walked over to the movie theater.

The movie we had chosen turned out to be pretty steamy and romantic, and I noticed that my mouth was hanging open, longing to be living the part. I wondered if Gary was feeling the same way. It wasn't easy having a platonic relationship with a person whom I was crazy about, especially in a movie like this. Gary now tells me that this was difficult for him too, because he was committed to Carla, and this movie kept reminding him of his attraction to me.

After the movie, Gary took me home and we promised to get together again soon. I wished him well in his relationship with Carla and told him that I was available to talk if he needed me. I then focused my attention on seeing Chad again.

On the following Saturday afternoon, Chad and his son joined us at one of Adam's track meets. We all had a pleasant time together.

Chad and I went to dinner and a movie that evening, and we had another great time. It felt good to be out with a decent, sensitive, affectionate man. I was really enjoying his companion-ship, and the feeling seemed to be mutual.

Later the following week, Chad called and told me that his old high school sweetheart had just moved back to L.A. and she wanted to date him again. Chad told me that he had always been crazy about her, and she had broken up with him years earlier to run off and marry someone else. Well, the marriage didn't work out, so she was coming back to Chad. I certainly understood and told Chad to just be careful and try not to get hurt again. We wished each other well, and promised to keep in touch. He did eventually marry her.

Chapter 14: GARY

The lectures

Later that month, my father signed me up for a group of lecture/discussions for young, single professionals. He felt that it would be a great way to meet some interesting people. I wasn't thrilled about going to this course alone. I told Gary about the course, and to my delight, he decided to take the course with me. Gary agreed to drive to my house and pick me up. He had recently proposed to Carla. So I asked if Carla would want to take the course with us. She was busy on those evenings, but Gary confessed much later that he was happy to attend with me alone because of the building tensions in his relationship with her.

Gary and I sat together for the lectures. Gary encouraged me to mingle with the other single men during the breaks, in the hopes that I might meet someone decent. I told him that I would love to meet someone just like him. He loved the compliment. Little did he know that I wanted him. Or, maybe he did.

At this time I wasn't dating anyone, and I actually felt a sense of relief. I again felt like I had enough of dating for a while. If a decent man came my way, that would be wonderful, but I wasn't desperate and certainly wouldn't settle for just anyone. So for the time being, I spent my time with my children and girlfriends, and was quite content.

Gary was busy making plans for his marriage to Carla. Gail and I were planning to attend his wedding together. Gary still seemed to have some reservations about this woman, and I just hoped that he would make the right decision.

The month of May proved to be very interesting. Gail met a fabulous man, who seemed like the man of her dreams. I was so excited for her. We made plans to have dinner together the following Saturday night, and I couldn't wait to hear all the details.

We begin to date

That Thursday night, Gary called. I hadn't talked to him for a while, so I was thrilled to hear from him and curious to know how things were going with his engagement. I was surprised when he told me that he had decided that she was not the right woman for him. There were continuing legal problems with her divorce and she was turning out to be very demanding in ways that were totally inappropriate. There were questions about priorities and commitment levels, previously left unspoken, but now coming to the surface. It was her way or no way, so they broke up.

He was pretty upset. I was positive that she would come back to him when she realized what she had lost. Gary didn't agree. He asked me if I was free Saturday night for dinner. I had plans with Gail, but he was more than welcome to join us. He agreed, and I was delighted. I hoped to help him feel better.

Gail and Gary met me at my townhouse, and then we all drove together in Gary's car to the restaurant. Gail told us all about her wonderful new boyfriend, Carl, who she later married, and we were both so happy for her. Gary told us about the conflict with Carla, which caused him to change his decision on the marriage, and we both agreed that he was right this time. They were very clearly wrong for each other, although I told him once again, that she would come back to him when she realized what she had lost. Gary still didn't agree with me.

Following dinner, Gail said that she had to get home. We drove back to my place, and after we said goodbye to Gail and saw her off, Gary asked me if I'd like to go somewhere for coffee. So we got back into the car and drove to a nearby trendy French restaurant. While we were waiting for our coffee and dessert, Gary said to me, "You know how I said that we could never date because I could never handle three boys?"

I answered, "Yes."

"Well," he went on, "why don't we give it a try."

I couldn't believe what I was hearing. Gary was asking me

to date him. I repeated to him what I thought he was saying. He confirmed it. I was absolutely ecstatic, although tried not to show it.

After our dessert and coffee, Gary drove me home and when he kissed me passionately good night, it was as natural as if we had been intimate for years. We were meant for each other. I knew that I could give him what no other woman could. He was, and still is, a treasure, and I vowed never to stop appreciating him. He was my best friend, and soon he would be my lover. What could be better?

Gary asked me out the next weekend. He wanted to take me to a play in Westwood. I could hardly contain myself. All week I was on "cloud nine." The weekend came, and we had such a wonderful time. It was such a relief to finally be able to hold his hand and hug and kiss him. When he brought me home, he stayed for quite awhile. We had lots of catching up to do.

Two steps forward, one back

But a cloud hovered over my soaring mood. Gary told me that because he had just come out of the relationship with Carla, and still having separation anxiety, he felt that he should continue to meet other women for a while. He wanted to rule out a rebound situation and be sure that his feelings for me were real. I was devastated because, without a doubt, he was the right one for me, and we had both acknowledged that we had always had feelings for each other. Still, I had to go along with his wishes. He just wanted to be cautious and sure.

Gary continued to see me several times a week, and then he would have people fix him up with other women, or he would respond to an ad in one of the Singles magazines, mostly for coffee meetings only. He was always very honest with me, and always told me when he was going out with one of these other women. Afterwards, he would call me and tell me what he liked or didn't like about the woman. I tried to remain cool and collected, but inwardly, this all hurt very much.

One day Gary said to me that sometimes he asked himself why he was seeking out so much "hamburger," when he already had a "steak." I appreciated the compliment, although I wondered the same thing. There was nothing that I could do except to wait for Gary to get this business out of his system, with the hopes that he wouldn't meet anybody that he liked more than me.

One afternoon in mid-June, Gary paged me. When I returned his call, he sounded awful. I asked him what was wrong. My predictions had come true, and Carla had just come over to his house to try and get back together with him. He told her that it just wouldn't work between them. She became very upset and stormed off, under the assumption that he would change his mind. Gary was an emotional wreck. I felt badly for him, and told him to relax and we would get together later in the day. I commended him on how well he handled Carla, and reiterated to him that he had made the right decision in ending their relationship.

Gary and I made plans to have dinner the following Saturday evening, with **Rob**, another widower from our support group.

We arrived at the Crocodile Cafe a few minutes early. When we were seated, Gary suggested that I sit across from him, instead of next to him. When I inquired as to why he wanted this seating arrangement, he told me that if Rob were interested in possibly dating me, it would be easier for him to approach me, without thinking that I had anything going with Gary.

I couldn't believe Gary. I knew that he was trying to be diplomatic with me, since he was still seeing other women; but trying to play it fair this way, really backfired and hurt me.

I ended up sitting next to Gary, anyway.

In early August, one of my friends told me that a colleague of her husband was coming into town from New York to take care of some business. Knowing my situation with Gary, she asked if I would like to join them and the colleague, for dinner the following Friday night. She told me that he was a great guy and that I would have a lot of fun. Apparently, he had recently been divorced and was anxious to meet new people. I accepted, although my heart was still with Gary.

I called Gary that evening and told him about my Friday night invitation. He thought that it sounded great and he encouraged me to go and have a good time. I was a little disappointed with his enthusiastic attitude. What I wanted to hear was, "Don't go. I couldn't stand the thought of you with another man!" He subsequently told me that he was thinking just that, but wanted to be fair. Oh well. I was determined to have a good time.

I drove to the restaurant with my friends and met **Derek** there. He was warm, charming, and fascinating, and the evening was fabulous! He was a studio special effects director. I was truly taken with him. He was so kind and seemed truly interested in finding out all about me. He showered me with compliments and made me feel wonderful. It was no surprise when he asked me for my number and expressed a strong desire to see me again.

After arriving home that evening, I called Gary and told him about the dinner. When I said that Derek really liked me, Gary said that he wasn't surprised. Once again, this disappointed me. I had hoped that Gary would have shown just a little jealousy. Gary didn't feel that it was appropriate to express feelings of jealousy since he had dictated the open terms of our current dating situation.

After my call with Gary, my phone rang. It was Derek. He told me that he was in town until Sunday night, and he asked me out for Saturday afternoon and evening. I was quite flattered by his attention. I accepted his invitation for Saturday afternoon, but told him that I had other plans for the evening. Gary was taking me to the theater.

I made sure that the boys had plans for the day, and then anxiously awaited Derek's arrival. He came exactly on time, and we drove to a restaurant on the beach in Malibu. We had drinks, appetizers, and a fabulous lunch. We sat and talked for what seemed like hours. He was really a lovely, brilliant, romantic, man and I really enjoyed his company. When he drove me home, he told me that he was crazy about me and wanted to see me again before he had to leave for New York. Since I was busy that Saturday evening, he asked me to go out with him Sunday morning and afternoon. I had no other pressing plans, so I accepted.

Derek picked me up around 11:30 that Sunday morning, and we went for brunch and then to The Los Angeles County Museum of Art. Since his flight to New York that evening wasn't until 8:00, we had dinner together, as well. When he drove me home, he told me all of the things that I would have wanted to hear from Gary. He said that he thought that I was very special, and he said that he adored me. He said that he hated to leave me, and would find a way to come back soon. This was wonderful and so refreshing, since I felt like I hadn't been appreciated that vehemently in a long time.

I was very surprised that evening when Derek called me from the airplane, while en route to New York. He told me that he just couldn't get me out of his mind. He went on to say that he believed that he was falling in love with me. I told him to take it easy. All this infatuation with me could be the result of a rebound effect from his recent divorce. He told me that this was absolutely not the case. He said that his divorce might have been recent, but the marriage had been over long before, and he now knew exactly the type of woman he wanted, and I was that woman. Now that he had found me, he wasn't about to let me go. Somewhere deep inside I also thought his obsession with me might not be completely healthy, but I was enjoying this too much to pay my inner thoughts any real attention.

Once again, I was very flattered. I then remembered that he was talking to me for thirty minutes on the airplane cellular. We ended the conversation, and he hesitantly said goodbye and told me that he would call me when he got in to New York.

Boy, was I confused. I loved the way Derek treated me, but my heart was still with Gary. Only time would tell. I was feeling a little depressed because a few weeks later, Gary was leaving me for a two-week vacation with his daughters. They were going back east to visit with relatives. I volunteered to drive them to and from the airport.

True to his word, Derek called when he arrived back in New York. In fact, he called me three and four times a day. He told me that he wanted to come to L.A. to see me as soon as possible. He said that he could come for a week and combine a little business with a lot of pleasure. The best time to come was when Gary was away. Then I wouldn't be so lonely, and I could really get to know Derek and evaluate whether he would make a good partner in life for me. I was feeling very frustrated with Gary's inability to fully commit to me, so I felt that I deserved to give myself options.

I saw Gary and the girls off on a Thursday night, and Derek flew into Los Angeles to be with me the following Sunday. That week was exhausting! Derek was so attentive, sometimes even too attentive. I needed time to breathe. He even took me with him when he had to go to the Hollywood studio. He was wonderful with my boys, and took them to the studio sets. The boys thought that he was awesome. They loved all of the excitement, and responded affectionately to Derek. We were busy from morning till late night.

A few times that week, when I arrived home at night, there were messages from Gary. As the week progressed, Gary's messages would get more frequent. Finally, since I very seldom was around at an opportune time to return his calls, he left a message saying that he wondered if I still existed. It was evident that he was getting quite frustrated with me. He knew that something was happening.

Finally, after setting my clock to get up early one morning, I called Gary in New Jersey. Hearing his voice made me acutely aware of how much I missed him. He asked me where I had been all week. I wasn't ready to tell him about my relationship with Derek, so I told him that I had just been really busy. I could tell that he was not convinced. He had told all of his relatives about me, and how much he liked me. This made me feel good. When we said goodbye, I told him that I would be waiting at the airport for him and the girls when they returned.

When I was with Derek later that day, he told me that he had some great news. He was able to extend his trip and leave, unbeknownst to him, on the same flight on which Gary was returning.

I just couldn't believe this! Well, at least I had some time to think about how I was going to handle this. I certainly wasn't ready to see both Gary and Derek together.

The rest of the week was hectic, but fabulous. I had such a great time. My friends were thrilled for me. They said that I deserved to be wined and dined and appreciated for the wonderful woman that I was. They always knew how to make me feel good.

When it was almost time for the week to end, Derek proposed to me. He told me that he loved me more than anything, and he wanted to spend the rest of his life with me. He told me that he wanted to take care of me totally so all that I would have to worry about, was writing my children's stories, a passion that I wanted to fulfill. Derek put me up on a pedestal and vowed that he would make me the happiest, most content woman in this world. What could I say? He said all of the things that I dreamed someone would say to me one day.

I told Derek that I would need some time to think about this proposal. I needed to know how Gary truly felt about me. I was resentful of Gary in a way, because he couldn't decide if he wanted to spend the rest of his life with me or not, and here Derek wanted me forever, with no doubts. He said, "I know something good when I see it and I'm not about to let you go!" I was very confused. I was in love with Derek's words, but I wasn't sure if I loved him, especially so quickly. I always loved Gary, but if Gary wasn't sure about me, then why should I give up Derek?

I was getting more and more apprehensive about the airport situation. Luckily, just as the day arrived, Derek came to pick me up, and told me that he was able to extend his stay another day, so he wouldn't be going on Gary's flight after all. Boy, did I sigh with relief.

Gary and the girls came in from New Jersey, as planned, and I was there to meet them. Gary looked great and I realized how much I missed him. Why couldn't he have been the one to have proposed to me?

I drove them home, and after helping them get settled, I told Gary that I had to leave. Gary walked me out and said that he wanted to see me that evening. I really wanted to be with him, but it was Derek's last evening in town, and I promised to be with him. I told Gary that because of his trip, I thought he would be too exhausted to get together that night, so I made other plans. Gary was visibly disappointed, and I felt terrible, especially considering Gary's perception skills. We did make plans to get together the next evening.

Derek picked me up that evening, and we joined some of his friends at a Mexican restaurant. We ordered Margaritas, dinner, and had a great time; however, Gary was constantly in the back of my mind. I had a real dilemma.

Derek and I said our goodbyes, and he pleaded with me to give him a positive response to his proposal. He even swore that he would relocate here in Los Angeles to make things easier for me. He told me that he wouldn't leave me alone until I gave him an answer. Once again, he called me over and over from the plane while in flight to New York.

Finally I told him not to call anymore that evening because

I was not going to be home. He became very worried and asked me where I was planning to go. I told him that I was spending the evening with Gary. He wasn't happy, to say the least.

Gary finally commits

I met Gary at his house, because I told him that we needed to talk. The girls were not at home, so we had our privacy. There was a tension between us that we had never experienced before. I knew that I was sending out weird vibes. Gary and I were so in tuned to each other, that we could sense immediately when something wasn't right. We sat in the family room, and I proceeded to tell Gary about Derek.

"Gary," I said. "Remember the man that I met when I went out to dinner with my friends?"

Gary acknowledged that he remembered.

"Well," I went on, "he liked me so much that he came to visit me while you were away."

Gary said, "Oh, well that explains why I could never reach you." He didn't look too pleased.

"Anyhow," I went on, "we spent quite a bit of time together and he has asked me to marry him."

Gary was furious. He questioned me as to how I could even consider marrying someone that I had only known for a few weeks.

I told him that Derek was just so good to me, that Derek truly adored me and assured me that I was the most important part of his life. I told him that Derek wanted to take all my worries away and take care of me. I told him that Derek loved me.

Gary immediately stood up and shouted, "I love you, and I have always loved you! I want to do all the things that Derek promises, and more! You're making a big mistake if you go with him. His love could never be as sincere as mine!"

I was shocked. Gary really did love me. I couldn't believe what I was hearing. I told Gary that I was always madly in love with him, but I just didn't think that he loved me. Derek was telling me all the things that I was starving to hear. I went on to tell Gary that I was terribly frustrated. I needed and wanted to feel loved. The dates that he continued to go on were hurting me terribly, and I finally met a man who thought I was the most important person in his life, and he wanted to devote his life to me.

Gary warned me that I would be making the biggest mistake of my life if I married Derek. Gary said that he truly loved me and he would gladly give up these other dates and just see me exclusively from now on. He wanted to get our families together on a daily basis to see if we all got along. If things went well, we would be heading towards marriage.

I accepted this plan, because I loved Gary and really did want to spend the rest of my life with him. It felt wonderful to hear him profess his love for me, and with such passion. Gary is very cautious about whatever he does, and he doesn't make snap decisions. He takes his time and explores all his options. I was going to try and be patient.

Now I had the sad task of telling Derek. When I told him, he just wouldn't accept my decision. He called and called and wrote letter after letter telling me that he loved me and couldn't live without me. After many conversations, he finally, very reluctantly, had no choice but to accept my decision. He was devastated, and I felt terrible.

I spoke to my Bettylou about what was going on. She thought that Derek sounded terrific. She didn't know Gary very well, but I had told her about how hurt I had been when Gary continued to date other women while dating me. She told me that she hoped that I was making the right decision. She said that it would be a real shame to lose Derek, if things didn't work out with Gary, and I deserved so much more than I was currently getting from Gary. She felt that beyond a doubt, Derek would treat me as a precious treasure; however, she would be supportive of whatever made me happy.

So, the terms of our dating changed, and Gary and I became more committed to one another. The children all seemed to get along okay. Gary was slowly adjusting to the boys. They were much more active and challenging than the girls had been, and he was getting used to their ways.

Everything was going quite well. Gary took me to Newport Beach for a weekend in October, and we had a magical time. It was our first time away together. During Thanksgiving vacation, both of our families shared a trip to San Diego. We once again had a great time. We came back from San Diego on Saturday night, left the children with Ellie, Gary's older daughter, and Gary took me to Pasadena for the night. We stayed at a beautiful hotel, and the next morning we went to the annual Harvest Festival, where we began to shop for holiday gifts together.

We were becoming more and more attached to one another, and if it was possible, I was falling more deeply in love with him. Every moment that we were together just affirmed that I had made the correct decision.

The holidays soon arrived, and both of our families had the most wonderful time together. It was a time of mutual love, giving, and sharing, and we all felt truly united. I just knew that this union was going to work. We were all so good together.

In October we had a group photograph taken of all seven of us. The photo came out great, and for Christmas, Gary gave me a beautiful round charm holder, which when opened, unfolded with a picture of Gary and each of the five children, which Gary had cleverly prepared from the group photo. I was so touched. This was an encouraging sign that Gary wanted this relationship to last for good.

Gary made plans to take our families up the coast to Monterey during the week between Christmas and New Year's Eve. He even rented a van so that we could all travel together. We had another fabulous time, and the bond was sealing tighter between our two families.

As New Year's Eve arrived, I was becoming very excited. We were entering a new year and I wondered what Gary had in mind. He made reservations at a very romantic restaurant, and I could hardly wait to celebrate with him. We had so much to look forward to. Everything seemed to be going so well.

A setback

While getting ready for the evening, I received a very disturbing call from my girlfriend, Candy. Adam had been with her son, having spent the previous night at their house. The boys had been fooling around near the local elementary school, and did some damage to the grounds. Candy said that we had to get together immediately and talk about what had happened.

I couldn't believe what I was hearing. I also knew that if Gary found out about this, he probably wouldn't want to marry me. What horrible timing. Just when I was so happy, something like this had to happen to spoil it all. I cried to Candy, telling her of my predicament. She felt badly and apologized for the boys not being supervised well enough. I didn't blame her. These boys were old enough to use proper judgment, and we both decided that they had to suffer their own consequences for their irresponsible actions. Candy was in the middle of chemotherapy for breast cancer. This was all she needed. She needed me there with her.

Oh, how I dreaded telling Gary about this. I had to tell him right away, because Candy wanted me to come over to discuss what had happened. This would change our evening plans. I was absolutely devastated. I called Gary and told him what had happened. He was not pleased, to say the least. He did say that he would come right over and accompany me to Candy's house.

It was a stressful evening, although we got through it. We never made our dinner reservation, but we did have a small meal late in the evening. After dinner, we welcomed the New Year together, and hoped for better times ahead. He did not propose to me, although that had been his plan. After this episode with Adam, I knew that he wouldn't. Suddenly, the future held so many doubts.

Adam was remorseful and he personally apologized for what had happened. This whole situation really freaked Gary out, because his girls rarely got into any trouble at all. I explained to him once again, that boys were different and their issues were different than girls' issues. He listened, but it would take him awhile before he would be able to accept these added complications to his life. I understood his apprehension, yet hoped that he loved me enough to overcome it.

With the arrival of this new year and my renewed happiness, I was finally emotionally ready to open Sandy's closet and go through his clothes. I kept many of the nicer articles of clothing for the boys and for myself. The other items went to Marta and her family, and to charity. Sandy was gone, and I was now able to completely say goodbye, and look towards my future, hopefully with Gary.

Before I knew it, March had arrived, and it was time to make summer plans for the children. Last December I had hoped that our summer plans would have included a union between our families. Now, I had to plan as I did all the previous summers. Once this was done, I felt very depressed, wondering what the future would hold.

Gary's proposal

The last day of March, 1995, was a Friday night. Gary told me to dress nicely for dinner at the Inn of the Seventh Ray. It was a lovely, romantic restaurant deep in Topanga Canyon. When we arrived at the restaurant, we were escorted to a beautiful table, where Gary immediately ordered two glasses of wine. When the wine arrived, he held up his glass to make a toast. I held my glass up to his. After making our usual toast, Gary said, "Now I want to make another toast." As he looked deeply into my eyes, he said, "To the rest of our lives together."

I said, "What does that mean?"

Gary said, "I'm asking you to marry me!"

I said, "Would you repeat the question?"

He did, and I was thrilled. My dreams had finally come true.

We were so excited we could hardly eat our dinner. We went back to Gary's house and immediately called our parents. They were all thrilled for us. Then we told the children, as they came home. They were also ecstatic! They would finally have a complete family again.

We wanted to get married as soon as possible. The boys and I would be moving into Gary's house. We chose July 30, 1995 as the wedding date. This would give us adequate time to plan the wedding and the move out of the townhouse.

Sandy's family was thrilled for us and Gary's first wife's family was also thrilled. They both knew how much each of us had suffered, and they were happy to see that we both found happiness again. We would continue to have a very close relationship with our extended families.

The plans were progressing well, and we were so excited. This wedding was going to be the happiest day in our lives. I was so thankful and so blessed. I found the man of my dreams and he was going to be my husband.

Another complication

But there are always complications. The middle of April, I had a slight setback. One Thursday evening as I went into the boys' room to kiss them good night, I leaned down to kiss Adam. He was lying on his stomach, and I presumed that he was asleep. As I leaned down to kiss the back of his head, I startled him, and he threw his head back, smashing into my nose. Gary came running into the room, having heard the horrible crack as my nose broke.

The next day, after seeing the doctor, it was confirmed that I had a double fracture. The bridge of my nose was broken, as well as the septum. These breaks would require surgery, which was scheduled the following day.

How could this be happening? It seemed that every time something good happened to me, something else would happen to complicate things. Here I was to be married in just a couple of months. How was I going to look?

I had the surgery on Monday. My parents and Gary were at the hospital. They were all so wonderful and so attentive to me. After the surgery, Gary took me home, and for the next week, he and Robyn, his younger daughter, moved in with us, so that he could take care of me. Gary was unbelievably good to me. After getting the children off to school, he would shop for me and make sure that all my needs were met. He was amazing. I was, and still am, the luckiest woman in the world. My parents were also wonderful, as were all of my friends.

After about a week, I started to feel better, and resumed most of my usual routine. The doctor said that it would take a while for all of the swelling to go down, but he felt that I would be back to normal by the wedding date. Oh, how I hoped that he was right.

Continuing the wedding plans

We continued with the planning of the wedding. We chose Braemar Country Club in the mountains above Tarzana, for the wedding and luncheon, which my parents gave. They were thrilled for the both of us, and they really thought that Gary was right for me. My mother and I had great fun planning the details that would make this wedding perfect.

After most of the details were decided, I now had the wonderful task of picking out a wedding dress. It didn't take long to find. Ronna came with me. We went to a Victorian Bridal Shop. When I walked into the store, it was as if the dress was waiting there just for me. It was really unbelievable! The dress caught my eye immediately. It was made of white lace, which went down to the ankle. I also chose beautiful white lace shoes to match. I asked the florist to make my headpiece of baby white roses. The dress, though elegant, was very simple, and not nearly as ostentatious as a traditional wedding gown.

Gary decided that he would wear a gray morning coat tuxedo. The boys would wear black tuxedos and the girls would wear white dresses. Everything was going to be beautiful!

Gary and I met several times with Dr. John Sherwood, who would perform our wedding ceremony. He wanted to get to know us better and talk about the trials and tribulations of a blended family. He had also been widowed and remarried. We just knew that this wedding was going to be magical. We were so excited.

My sister-in-law, Sheila, gave me a beautiful wedding shower at a lovely restaurant. All of my girlfriends came, and it was a day to remember. My future in-laws were also in town to attend the party. Of course, my parents were there as well.

Sheila was wonderful. She was so happy for me, yet I knew that she was feeling sadness, too. This wasn't easy for her. I had been married to her brother, and now I was beginning a new life with a new husband. We vowed to remain close, and we are to this day. She may have lost a brother, but she gained a terrific brother-in-law.

Invitations went out and we were thrilled with the response. Nineteen family members from Gary's first wife's family were traveling from all over the country to come to our wedding. My aunts, uncles, and cousins from all over were coming as well. Sandy's family wouldn't have missed it for the world. Our friends were ecstatic. They had seen us at rock bottom, helped build us back up again, and now they were ready to come and help us celebrate the beginning of our new life together. We could hardly wait for the big day to arrive.

The wedding was set to begin at 11:00 on Sunday morning, July 30th. Out of town relatives started arriving on Friday. This gave Gary and me a little time to become acquainted with each other's families and extended families. We were both truly blessed. The families were wonderful, and we were both thrilled to be accepted with so much love. My future in-laws were and still are generous, loving, and kind.

On Saturday night Gary's parents hosted a dinner for the out of town guests. The most beautiful toasts were made to us. I felt as if I was in a dream. I couldn't believe that life could be this good. I couldn't wait for our marriage to begin.

The previous week, the boys and I moved from the townhouse into Gary's house in Calabasas. This meant that the boys would be attending new schools in September. They were so happy with their new dad, sisters, and new home, and they were excited to be attending new schools. It didn't appear that they would have any difficulty adjusting to a new life. I just knew that I had done well for them. If Sandy was up there watching, he would be so happy for us. We would finally be a complete family, and happy again.

The wedding ceremony

As the wedding ceremony began, the beautiful, spiritual music of Enya was played. As my father walked me down the aisle, I looked all around me. Ahead of me, I saw the canopy with my future husband waiting for me, and all of our children and parents up there as well. On both sides of me sat all of my wonderful friends, Gary's friends, and our families. There wasn't a dry eye in the room. These people had come so far with us, and they were all here to rejoice in our newly found love and happiness. My feelings totally overwhelmed me. As my father kissed me, and turned me over to Gary, I was home free. This was where I belonged. I found my true soul mate in life. I was overwhelmed with emotion. I could see that Gary was, as well. We were both crying, and the ceremony had not even begun.

The ceremony was magnificent. We couldn't have hoped for a better start in our new lives together. It was the most beautiful, personal, appropriately funny, touching, and emotional wedding that I had ever witnessed, and it was OUR wedding.

Following the ceremony, we had a fabulous party. We had a great Deejay, who played all of the music that we had requested, and he really kept the party lively. We partied until the very end, and we enjoyed every second of it. It was the happiest day of our lives.

I was now Mrs. Gary Young. My life was also enriched by two wonderful daughters, two fabulous in-laws, and a lovely extended family. What could be better?

My in-laws had volunteered to stay with the children while Gary and I went up to Santa Barbara and Big Sur in northern California, for our honeymoon.

The honeymoon

We drove home from the wedding, quickly changed, and drove up the coast to The Simpson House in Santa Barbara. It was a lovely, romantic, bed and breakfast inn. Here we spent our first night of marriage in our own little cottage.

The next morning, after a gourmet breakfast on the patio of our cottage, we left for Big Sur. While driving up the California coast, Gary and I reflected on our lives, and decided to write this book. Everyone who came in contact with us felt that our story could give support to people, and we wanted to share our experience. We wanted people out there to know that when tragedy strikes, it doesn't always mean that life is over. Many times happiness can be found again. It may take awhile, but it can be found. And life can even be better than it was before.

We arrived in Big Sur and checked into The Ventana, the exclusive inn hidden away high up in the mountains overlooking the Pacific Ocean. As we looked below us, we could see a blanket of clouds separating us from the rest of the world. We felt as if we were in Heaven.

After we arrived in our magnificent suite, we relaxed, and then had a delicious, romantic dinner in the Ventana dining room. After dinner, we relaxed in the outdoor hot tubs, while gazing at the stars. Even though a blanket of clouds lay below us, above us, it was clearer than we had ever seen skies before. This was just a continuation of the magic that was following us everywhere.

After the hot tubs, we came back to our suite, opened a bottle of champagne, and sat outside on our patio sipping champagne, counting shooting stars, and reflecting on our past.

The past four years have been painful, and I have come a

long way, learning many lessons. My spiritual and emotional growth, have made me a stronger woman and I am forever grateful for the good in my life today. I am one of the happiest and luckiest women in the world, and I will never take anyone or anything for granted for the rest of my life.

EPILOGUE: OUR STORY
since yesterday

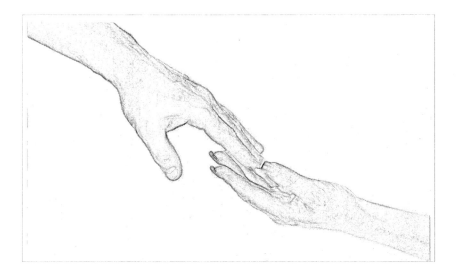

One of the facts of life is that every lovely dream realized has a reality attached to it. Some may call it the "fine print," or the "anti-escape clause." The idyllic setting of our honeymoon at Big Sur was so compelling that we returned the following year. Since we were not trying to rerun the events and emotions of the honeymoon, we enjoyed the second visit thoroughly.

It seemed like we had been living in a hyper-reality during the time when the difficulties of grieving were being worked out. In contrast, the honeymoon seemed more like a perfect fantasy. But if we were living in a fantasy world during the honeymoon, reality regained its foothold the minute we returned home. We wanted the honeymoon to last forever, and who doesn't? And in many ways, it has lasted through the years of marriage. But there is that reality...

We are plodding our way through an interesting mix. We still feel like newlyweds because we have learned to cherish every moment and never take each other for granted. At the same time we are dealing with the interactions, reactions and adjustments, and the quest for a clearer focus on the changing issues that the children have. Life is not boring, with guitar, singing, drums, dance, soccer, drums, soccer, soccer, football, school, scouts, competing weekend transportation requirements, our professional lives, drums, drums, drums...and soccer. Five children. Two girls and three boys. No, not the Brady Bunch. If we want to be numerically correct, it would be the Partridge Family. However, it really isn't that, nor is it My Three Sons, Leave It to Beaver or Lassie, but a combination of the worst and best of those and other shows, plus a little Mission Impossible and Lost in Space.

The interactions with the children sometimes take us to wit's end and even further. We share anger, rage, frustration, headaches, bewilderment, and reconciliation. The mix is very interesting. Ellie, Robyn, Jamie, Adam and Jordan each have strong personalities, each have a complex and interesting sense of humor.

Each has an interesting and challenging take on reality, and each have impressive talents such as music, soccer, skateboarding, dance, studies, art, debating, and the list goes on. At this moment we have four teenagers and one adult, so we are dealing with new drivers, college, and (gulp) serious boy or girl friends.

Gary found out, as expected, that boys are different from girls, and that he is again young enough to brandish a squirt gun. And Kathy found out that girls are different from boys and that girl talk is more fun than ever. Gary's quiet past is now a noisy present. The decibels are high. Adam is a talented guitarist and writer, and Jordan is an exceptional drummer (it was Gary's idea!) in a new band that is really catching on fast. Robyn has held several offices in a rare coeducational high adventure Scout troop, she had the lead in her school play, civic awards, and so forth. Ellie and Jamie are at school, studying design and aviation respectively, in which they have extraordinary talent and energy. We also have lots of spirited sibling rivalry and acting out. There is a truly eclectic mix of talent and frustration. Most people would call that normal in a house with five children approaching, in, and just outside their teen years, especially in a blended family. And the ground rules and power issues are many.

Kathy and I found the magical hours between 11:00 P.M. and 2:00 A.M. to be the best time for us to have quality time. It is quiet, and we can talk, make love like very tired newlyweds, giggle, complain, and have forbidden snacks. Then up at 6:00 A.M. We don't know why we frequently feel tired. This routine continues, with appropriate but not frequent enough rest moments, naps, and vacations.

Our time together still feels like a honeymoon. Yes, the five children bring that into a reality when we least expect it. But, believe it or not, we usually do get the 11:00 P.M. to 2:00 A.M. time clearly to ourselves.

In our immediate future, we have lots of graduations, lots of drivers, lots of college students, lots of weddings and God willing, lots of grandchildren.

Reality? Then it would be fair to point out that we will never forget what happened to us, and that we know that it could happen again, at any time. The gift is that we have learned to appreciate what we have in a more heightened way than before, more directly, having learned this lesson the hard way. We do not squander our moments together, and we take more time than ever to be with each other and appreciate each other. Part of that is maturity, but much of that is the painful lesson of not having had enough time with out first spouses and sometimes squandering the time that we did have. Our deceased spouses are still with us, with love, with fond remembrance, sometimes with anger, but not forgotten. We do not dwell on our losses or our tragedy. It did happen, and it contributed to shaping our lives, and will continue to do so. There is, after all, room for everyone in our hearts. And that includes our first spouses, five children, all of our extended families, and of course, our friends.

It took time figuring out the mechanics of this new family, and the process is reformulated daily. And the grocery bills! But we have what we wanted, a life with love and tenderness, not alone, not dwelling on the past or trying to reinvent it, nor erase it. We still cry occasionally when something hits a chord, and usually both at the same time. But we also laugh together. We are growing more alike daily, and even though in many ways we are still acting like newlyweds, people tell us that we are like a couple who have been together for a long time. Well, it has been a long time, if you include the three years of friendship, having met in 1991.

We are told that the years with the children will go quickly. Our lesson has re-taught us what we already knew, that included in the madness of parenting are beautiful moments that also should not be squandered. And after the children have left the nest, we hope to be there for each other.

Our lesson was learned the hard way, and it hurt. We are limping a bit from that, and we see frequent reminders that the rug can still be pulled out from under us, but we have what we have, and it is now, and we have chosen to be survivors.

APPENDIX A:

YOUNG WIDOWS AND WIDOWERS FACE OTHER ISSUES

We experienced a world upside down and backwards until we made sense of it and began the trials and tribulations of normalization. But there are many more issues faced by young widows and widowers. Through our involvement in our support group, first as members of the group and later as co-facilitators, plus our interaction with many young widows and widowers, we shared many additional questions, problems, and issues.

No two people are alike, of course, and there are still more issues than this list encompasses. So you may want to look at this list as a cursory guide to the problems that you may have encountered. Each subject below could easily be the theme of an entire book. We do not mean to gloss over these important subjects, but we did feel that it was important to acknowledge them. We experienced some of these and escaped the clutches of some. Since the solution to these problems takes more space and time than any complete book, you might want to use these topics as the start of a discussion about these and other issues, geared to your specific situation.

If there is no support group where you live, it might be possible to discuss issues with your friends, your family, your clergy, psychologists, or you may want to find an expert and start a support group. This person does not have to be a psychologist, but he or she should have more than the basic understanding of the field, and of people.

Certainly, many of the issues in this book apply equally to younger and older people.

Social Security defines a young widow or widower as a person between the ages of eighteen and fifty. Contact Social Se curity. You and your children may be eligible for assistance.

> **survivor's benefits. www.ssa.gov** or
> **www.ssa.gov/reach.htm** or call **1-800-772-1213**

Changes. Many people experience **sleep and appetite changes**, leading to loss or gain in weight and often **sleep deprivation**. Sleep deprivation is hard to avoid, but it has an insidious effect on long and short-term health. Some people are pressured into **relocating** to other cities, closer to family, but away from familiar territory. This also becomes a problem for the children. Any **Illness**, whether contracted by the parent or a child, or both, compounds the difficulties without the spouse for support or motivation. It is often difficult to fall back into **old habits and patterns**, since your life has been radically changed. This can be an opportunity to find **new stimulus**, leading to new patterns and a re-definition, rediscovery, or repositioning of some of the old patterns. You will be called to do **tasks** that you never in your wildest dreams though you would have to do. Wearing many different hats is both a challenge and an opportunity.

Tasks. Single parents are often called to do tasks that were formerly accomplished by the deceased spouse. The long list ranges from driveway repair, to car repair, to managing finances.

Events that can throw us off. Some widows and widowers find the **change from daylight savings time** to standard time a depressing moment. There is more darkness of course, and the idea of additional darkness is depressing to some, and it is also the lonely time. **Any anniversary**, whether the anniversary of the death, or a birthday, or a holiday, or even the anniversary of an engagement or event, all can throw us off, often when we least expect it.

Absentmindedness seems to plague all of us. People lose the key to their safety deposit box at the worst possible time, house keys, car keys, even cars when we forget where we parked at the shopping center.

Insurance carriers are sometimes reluctant to pay until we can prove things that are already a matter of public record. Some people are saddled with **hospital bills** totaling well into the millions. The insurance contracts might have to be fought in a costly manner, with the specter of a losing battle affecting the children's welfare.

How our spouses died. This is as varied as the individual circumstances surrounding the grief period. People in our support groups experienced disease, murder, suicide, drunk drivers, vacation accidents, bizarre accidents, flu, illnesses contracted in foreign countries, industrial accidents, heart attacks, terrorist attacks, and even a SIDS-like condition. One gentleman who was married to a younger woman, developed terminal cancer but died in a boating accident while on vacation, while trying to live as fully as possible during his remaining days. The family **blamed** the young wife, irrationally. But emotion is always irrational. Bereavement is irrational, but at the same time all too real.

Anger. It is common to feel anger when a spouse dies. Perhaps this person did not take care of his or her health properly. Perhaps he took too many life-threatening chances. Maybe he was in **denial** of an illness and lost valuable time in that process. But as irrational as emotion is, we might simply be angry that the spouse left us. We are left to fend for ourselves, and we are forced **to do and learn to do things in which we have no interest**, experience, aptitude, or time. And we can be angry with ourselves for **things that we did or did not do or say**. We can be angry with ourselves because **we are still here and they are not**; that we can live to enjoy life and see our children grow, and they cannot. We can be angry with family for **saying the wrong thing**, or doing something **insensitive**, or for giving either **inadequate or too much attention**. We can be angry with **friends who abandon** us because they are frightened, or are uncomfortable in our presence. We can be irrationally angry with a bank teller who takes a little too long. **Patience** is a skill that often needs to be re-acquired. Kathy's boys experienced such virulent anger that they sometimes told her that they wish she had died instead of Sandy, or that they thought that she was stupid for marrying a man who smoked. In the case of suicide, it is not uncommon to experience anger. Anger is normal, and can be a healing vent. We try not to deny our emotions, since there are so many emotions, at this time.

Words and Phrases that we hear: Words can be healing but often are maddening. Here is a phrase that we have heard often, but as well-intentioned as it is, we prefer not to blame God for our misfortune. "**God never gives you more than you can handle**." In Gary's play, *Interruptions*, this phrase is criticized by a very strong woman whose husband just died, leaving her with a family full of major illnesses, including her own cancer. She says, " I can handle what I've been dealt. But God didn't cause it, and there IS a limit. And I'm right there." Kathy and I sometimes heard, "**You're lucky he died**," spoken by a few people undergoing ugly divorces. As understandable as a divorced person's anger might be, we are NOT lucky our spouses died. "**I lost my wife**." Gary never liked that phrase, even though he accidentally used it a few times. Being the literal person that he is, he did not feel that he had lost *Kathie*. That phrase sounds trivial compared to what she and Gary really went through. She was still with him in a very significant way, even though not in a corporeal sense.

Idealizing the dead spouse. We often tend to place the deceased spouse on a celestial pedestal. For that time, he or she is remembered as perfect and unreachable by any worldly standard. This is normal and healthy for a while. When we begin to remember the funny, sad, irritating moments, we begin to remember this person more fully, and we have a tool for recovery.

What do we miss the most? An endless list would include sharing in general, talking all night until you fall asleep in mid-*non sequitur*, sex or a nurturing human touch, sharing a bath, sharing a dessert, laughter, sleep, free time, the deceased person's scent, our past life, and more. Sometimes, in a strange way, we miss the unwelcome tumult and attention surrounding the death. The special talents that the deceased spouse brought to the relationship, whether it was humor, or cooking, or sports can be missed greatly, as can cold feet under the sheets, dandruff, and bickering.

The protagonist, Bob, in Gary's play, *Interruptions*, missed bounding out of bed and giggling in the morning, until he realized that he hadn't done this before his wife died. Logic seems to go out of the window because so much of our life is consumed with grief.

Quirks. When a spouse dies, we miss them, but we also miss some of the quirks that they brought into the relationship. Some of the quirks were amusing and some were irritating, but most of the widows would gladly accept a return of the irritation if the spouse could return. Some quirks, of course, are not missed, especially once we get past the idealized state and begin to see our deceased spouse as a human again. Their absence can actually give us a little freedom. One of the things that Gary needed badly after *Kathie* died, that she prohibited when she was alive, was the ability to watch TV late at night, or read with the light on. Especially after she died, it helped him channel my thoughts elsewhere, if only for brief periods of time.

What do we need that we are not receiving now? High on the long list would be cuddling, help with everything, support on every level, and the touch of another person, which can be alleviated on a certain level through massage. It can be very difficult to find adequate support from people who know how to communicate and help.

Panic attacks are common. They sometimes mimic heart attacks because some of the symptoms can be rapid heartbeat and hyperventilation, often with perspiration. In our support group many of us described our panic attacks. It was interesting seeing them from another perspective. Even if you know you're having a panic attack and nothing worse, it is still disquieting.

Hitting the bottom. Gary knew exactly when he hit the bottom of my long zombie state. Not everyone identifies the actual bottom, but it is a major relief to be on the upswing. It is as if he were in an immense emotional tunnel. When he hit bottom, he couldn't see the light at the other end, but he began to recognize that he was heading in that direction. As Zoltan says, in Gary's play, *Interruptions*, "There is one thing about hitting the bottom, you have no where to go but up, unless you stay at the bottom, of course."

Fears are magnified. Some of us are afraid to take the next step for fear that it will be a misstep and we'll get hurt, again. The absurdity of life is magnified. But it's worth taking the steps toward health and independence if you cherish the good moments and use them as a guide, a goal, and something of which you can be proud. Some people become frightened at night. Many miss being with someone, held tight, perhaps being sexual, but the prospect of a new partner can be frightening and alienating on many levels. We can experience the fear of more rejection. Death is sometimes emotionally felt as a kind of rejection. The prospect of dating, even on a platonic level, can be scary. We also fear losing another mate. We might worry that we will forget the sound of the deceased spouse's voice. Most bereaved parents fear dying and not being there for their children.

"Cant's." There are many new "cant's." Most of the "cant's" can be changed into an achievable goal, perhaps into, "Not yet, but I'm working on it." Solutions come with time and the willingness to do the hard work. Some temporary "cant's" include understanding our new identity, consistent sleep habits, dealing with money, and controlling food intake. It is not surprising that we forget many things, but many people have the opposite problem and wish that they could forget some of the details, and often there is a see saw combination of both.

Dislikes are many. Some people find that they hate God, usually a temporary but understandable state. Many have issues with psychiatrists, medical bills, police with bad news, HMO's, temper, and how insensitive some people can be. Friends and family of the deceased can be cruel, out of fear, sadness, ignorance of the facts, or sometimes for real reasons with bad timing. We can quickly become tired of hearing doctors say gloomy things. More positive voices can be found from people who have a better bedside manner or from people not directly involved with health care. Some spouses of suicide victims experience embarrassment.

They can't talk about suicide in front of young children and they hope that the children never hear from the outside. As glad as Gary was that he had learned how to cry, he also became angry that he needed to cry so much.

Peripheral losses add to the emotional mess. Such losses can include blame, leading to estrangement of sons, daughters, friends or other family members. It is possible for either men or women, to die prior to the birth of children. Financial loss can happen, due to lawsuits, medical bills, or bad investment advice. We feel sadness when we think of all the beauty that the spouse is missing, and little satisfaction that he or she is also missing ugly life events.

In-law rejection is one of the peripheral losses that sometimes cannot be helped. The in-law family is still attached since there was no separation due to divorce. Yet, many families find that the new circumstances cause them to drift apart, and that can feel like a loss for both sides. There are many cases where the in-laws blame the surviving spouse for the death, or they might blame each other for not doing more, whether this is a true assessment or a wrongful perception. This can be fleeting or it can even escalate into lawsuits. It can be difficult for in-laws to offer help because they are dealing with their own pain.

Unanswerable questions, including questions I'm not normally allowed to ask out-loud. Where did he put our check stubs? What does my deceased spouse think of the cemetery? I wonder how I would have conducted myself if this had happened to me. Does my spouse have a support group...over there? Is this all part of the "grand design?" Was there pain upon passing, or did calmness prevail? What were the last thoughts? Can he see me now? Will we ever communicate? Does he blame me for anything? In the case of an accident, did he know what was happening, or did he just "turn off?" Did he experience fear or concern for those left behind? Was it sad for him? Is it sad for him now? There are many more. The questions cannot be answered but we can learn to process them and accept. *In a well-run support group there are no forbidden subjects, allowing questions, discussions, and* *tears for any issue.*

What many people would have said about cancer: This is from Gary's play, *Interruptions*. Even though the character who says this is not *Kathie*, a few of the character traits are based on her. This is one thing that I am sure *Kathie* would have said to me if she had returned after her death. "It's no secret I hated going through what I went through. I hated what it did, does to you. It wasn't my fault, but I hated the fact that I caused pain. And while we're on the subject, I did NOT lose my battle with cancer. I WON the battle. Will you tell people that? I get really pissed off when I hear that. I won the battle! Ok, I lost the war, but everyone eventually loses the war. I managed cancer for six years and led a pretty damn normal life, considering. And almost beat it, if it hadn't been for the misdiagnosis, which is pointless to fret about now. So I won the battle."

What some of us would have like to have said. "You know that sweater you gave me for my forty-first birthday? I hated that sweater." "I'm crazy about you. I have been ever since you died." "I never thought I'd miss our bickering." "How could you do this to me." The complete list would be a mile long.

What we would love to be able to tell our spouse now. "I'm doing well now. I treasure what we had and I will never forget you." Now Kathy and Gary can share jokes and funny moments with each other. As newly bereaved people, these moments were not as meaningful because we could no longer share them with our spouse. We wish we could tell our spouse about world-shaking events, family events, and a million other things.

Something that can help: a diary. Many people keep a diary of daily events and emotional feelings. The diary is sometimes constructed to include letters to the deceased person, or it may take that form entirely. The cathartic effect varies from person to person, and not everyone has the time or patience for such an exercise. Diaries are often put aside and never read by the writer. A diary can become a very valuable legacy for your children and family who might benefit from its contents after you are gone.

Gary never kept such a diary. He was reality-challenged for a long time and he was not ready to put pen to paper. He felt as if I was in the state of emotional regurgitation, and that anything that he might write would be useless; that it was like a diary from a person with no life. He might have been temporarily correct about the lack of a full life at the time, but I was wrong about the value of writing. Kathy did not keep a diary but was lucky to have her family and friends with whom to vent her emotions. A diary does not have to be a critical masterpiece. It is a tool, to be used subjectively, with your own rules. The difference between *Loss and Found* and a diary, if Gary had written one, is that the diary is immediate and *Loss and Found* was put together considerably after the fact. We did not feel a cathartic response by writing *Loss and Found*, although it might be there subconsciously. Rewrites force us to re-live every event many times, often bringing pain, rather than catharsis. Kathy and Gary do receive strong emotional catharsis by knowing that we are helping people with this book, as well as when we talk and listen to bereaved people and help them directly, even if in a small way.

Hard truths. Everything having to do with the death is hard. For a while, every new problem causes us to switch gears and go into neutral if we are in a numb mode, or go backwards if we are coming to grips with reality. Ultimately, if we are fortunate, we can experience growth from this adversity. Things need to be put into perspective. That takes a bit of re-education. Anger, sadness, all of the emotions have their place, and all are normal, healthy responses, up to a point.

Blended families. Really, to do any justice to this subject requires an entire book, or more. A blended family is a very complicated juggling act, including day-to-day mechanics: Our way versus their way. Who goes where? Who does what? Why do we do that or don't do that? The struggle of one family's ground rules versus the other family's ground rules. Why am I stuck with a stepdad who is not as smart, not as athletic, not as mechanically minded, not as funny, not as nice, not as good looking as my real dad? What is he really going to do to me if I disobey?

Emotional conflicts combine anger, sadness, grief, and loneliness whether real or perceived, the "us against them" mentality, immaturity, patience, sibling interactions and new territorial issues, and the infinite variety of jealousies. The solution takes time and it requires creativity, patience, careful perception using as much objectivity as possible, and above all, listening!

A blended family where one or more spouse has been widowed has some problems and issues that are similar to a divorced family, of course, but most issues are different. Every blend has its own particular set of adjustments. Other blends include configurations where one or more parent is widowed, one or more parent is divorced and widowed, foster children, and the list goes on. Each mix, combined with individual family issues, makes a blended situation complicated.

Divorce versus widowhood. In one way, it might not really be overly important to compare the two, because most people do not experience both situations. But a comparison is inevitable in social situations, where we are aware that the two are distinctly different, affecting our interactions. Of course, there are obvious differences. A widow would rarely have to choose between "his" and "her" friends as one might in a divorce. But widows find that friends on both sides often change their attitudes and might even shun us because of fears and discomfort. In a widowed relationship, there is no "Ex" to torment, be tormented by nor to exchange positive ideas, nor comfort. There is no Ex to share the childrearing tasks, which can be both good and bad, depending on the dynamics. The politics between the children and the surviving parent can seem simpler without an Ex to consider, but the politics within the household can become very complicated due to the lack of a second parent, and the inevitable idealization of the deceased parent in comparison to the more earthly perception of the surviving parent. Neither divorce nor widowhood is better nor worse. Both conditions are usually very difficult in their own ways. This subject also requires its own book in order to even scratch the surface of the issues, and there are books that cover this.

Widowhood in a good marriage, versus a bad marriage. We have met many widowed people and almost all of them have grief issues, regardless of the success of the marriage. Even in a bad marriage, death represents a change imposed on the survivor. Not only do we recognize the death of a parent of our children, but also the death of any future with that person. There is no concrete chance for the two of you to right any wrongs, whether you feel that they were the fault of your spouse or yourself. Most of us have that issue to some extent, and idealization of the dead spouse can happen even after a bad marriage.

Some help that would have been good to receive. Gary eventually did receive information about Social Security but lost about six months due to his ignorance. He would have benefited by having some prior knowledge about arranging the funeral and all of the accompanying events. Gary should have surreptitiously contacted a hospice during the latter stages of *Kathie's* illness. She prohibited him from telling anyone, but he desperately needed help. A hospice would have helped him in confidentiality, and might even have helped her. If we had been given more time, the Wellness Community support groups could have been supportive and psychological counseling might have helped all of us. Gary did attend one meeting of the Wellness Community before *Kathie* died.

Shrines, both unintentional and deliberate. In Gary's play, *Interruptions*, the young widower, Bob, who is the focus of the play, has never washed the glass that his wife used before she went to the hospital for the last time. He takes a long time to come to the point of understanding that the glass has become a figurative receptacle of his sadness, and really was only a fragile reminder of his inability to move on to a healthy perspective. Many of us possess unintentional shrines by default. They are usually innocuous and inconspicuous, but they can play a big part in our recovery process, or lack thereof.

A shrine can take any form, from an intended item, such as a trophy that the deceased person earned, to the unconscious holding on to a check, written in the handwriting of the spouse, a sweatshirt with a special memory attached or especially a voice message on an answering machine. The answering machine seems to be one of the hardest changes to make. These items are not always a bad thing. Gary is pleased when he sees our girls wear some of *Kathie's* jewelry or her clothes. He still has her bronzed baby shoes, and he plans to keep them until his children ask for them, if that happens. The boys are now big enough to wear Sandy's clothing. We both have our photos and some of the artwork accumulated since the early years.

Shrines can be very positive during the process of normalization. They can serve a purpose unless or until they begin to unintentionally hold a person back from recovery. Like most things having to do with emotions, this is rarely a black and white issue.

Holding the emotion, denial. It's well known that men often have this problem. We know men who have taken up to ten years to begin processing their grief processing, and even to allow the thought that grief even existed. We also know some widows who deny their progress from a grieving state to a healthier place. The surviving spouse can also deny his or her own medical or nutritional needs until symptoms take over.

Why a support group might be all I need/Why I might need more than a support group. As Bob says in Gary's play, *Interruptions*, "I'm not depressed. I'm grieving. Grieving with extra sadness. It's allowed. Depression is a clinical state. I'm not clinical. I'm situational. My state was caused by an external event." *If* he is right, he may not need a psychologist or psychiatrist. A support group may be all he requires in order to normalize. For any individual, it might be difficult to determine. That is why we tried both. We found that the support group gave us the real world re-training that we needed, better than therapy. Others have found the opposite, or have benefited by a combination. We have known people to grieve so deeply that they required hospitalization. Our preference is to try a support group, if one is available, even if in combination with therapy. The group offers peer help and friendship, companionship, and problem solving in the real world.

Survivor guilt. Not only are we subject to guilt for being alive and potentially able to enjoy life, but there is a particular kind of guilt felt by a spouse who has survived a common disaster or accident. We often feel that it is unfair that our spouse died, and that it should have been us instead. This is magnified in a case where the deceased spouse gave up his or her own life to save the survivor. A level of survivor guilt can be felt even if the person is not family, but an entire world of reminders is present when the person is a very close friend, a relative, or a spouse. Many people who escaped the World Trade Center disaster are feeling this, along with Post Traumatic Stress Syndrome, and general depression. We would hope that another realization that might come out of such a disaster is the thankfulness that we are alive, with a new realization of the value and positive potential of life. But it takes some time to get to that point for many people.

Fatalistic attitude. It is not surprising that a person who has suffered the loss of a spouse, by any means, might feel fatalistic about life. "Why water our plants? They're eventually going to die anyway." Death is capricious and illogical. We see it coming and we ask why, or we don't see it coming and we also ask why. Difficult to avoid, especially at first, this is one of the many attitudes and emotions that we have to work on during the healing process.

Doing what my deceased spouse would have wanted. This can take time to work out. In a relationship, behavior parameters are set, allowing two people to live together in harmony. This can be as simple as the issue of watching TV until late at night while the other spouse is trying to sleep, to taking a vacation to a spot that your spouse would have wanted to see, but you are not as interested. You may find yourself cleaning the house, not the way you want to, but the way your spouse would have wanted. Messy house, cap on the toothpaste, a certain way to load the dishwasher, we sometimes find ourselves doing what would please our absent spouse, even if it is something unimportant to us, or something that we really do not want to do, just as a way to be a little closer in a figurative way. As usual, this can be a long list. Some of these behaviors are okay, because they have actually become a part of you through your relationship, but some might need to be scrutinized, so that you can find your own comfort level. Working through these behaviors rather than disowning them might provide beneficial therapy.

What do you think about how I managed things after you were gone? Understandable curiosity prompts this unanswerable rhetorical question. Rather than asking a question, this is really a statement evolving from, "I can't do it alone," to "I guess I have to manage," to "I guess I'm beginning to catch on," to "I'm proud of myself for being able to handle this challenge." We would love to receive a pat on the back from our deceased spouse, saying we're okay, and implying that they are okay as well, but since that does not present itself in a concrete form, we learn to be our own support.

Why there is no topic in this book entitled, "Mistakes." Even though we struggle through the whims of nature, we have chosen to be survivors. We have made many mistakes, some good and some bad, but we have learned from them and have become stronger, healthier individuals, concentrating on the positive rather than dwelling on the negative. We still have a lot to learn. There is no topic entitled, "Mistakes," because mistakes are a part of life, so we do our best, and we go on.

APPENDIX B:
Some very helpful resources:

AARP Widowed Persons Service (AARP WPS):
601 E Street, NW Washington, DC 20049 (202)434-2260
FAX: (202)434-6474   E-mail: griefandloss@aarp.org

WidowNet: www.fortnet.org/WidowNet

GriefNet: www.rivendell.org

Tom Golden: www.webhealing.com

The Compassionate Friends (TCF): www.compassionate-
friends.org Email:TCF_National@Prodigy.com
PO Box 3696 Oak Brook, IL 60522-3696 (630)990-0010
International support group-information, resources, friendship,
hope to bereaved parents, grandparents, siblings.

Hospice Foundation of America: www.hospicefoundation.org
2001 S Street, NW Washington, DC 2000
Phone: 202-638-5419 E-mail: hfa@hospicefoundation.org

National Self-Help Clearinghouse: www.selfhelpweb.org
Graduate School and University Center/CUNY Room 620-N
33 West 42nd Street New York NY 10036 212-642-2944

Parents Without Partners: www.parentswithoutpartners.org
1650 South Dixie Hwy, Suite 510,   Boca Raton, FL 33432-7461

TAPS (Tragedy Assistance Program for Survivors): www.taps.org
Support for those impacted by a death in the armed forces
2001 S Street, NW # 300 Washington, DC 20009
Phone: 800-959-TAPS FAX: 202-638-5312

The Dougy Center: www.dougy.org.
Support for children, teens, and families in Portland, Oregon

Shiva Foundation: www.goodgrief.org/
Dealing with grief, turning it into a positive, creative experience

RENEW Center for Personal Recovery: www.renew.com/
Judy Davidson, Ed.D. P.O. Box 125,
Berea, KY 40403 606-986-7878

ParentsDB: www.parentsdb.com/index_ie.asp
An interactive resource for Parents dedicated to Parenting

Young Widows online support group:
young-widows@egroups.com. Online dialog with people
everywhere. Sensitive, friendly group, but as with all online
activities, be careful how much personal information you offer.

Motherless Daughters ™ of Los Angeles:
http://www.motherlessdaughtersbiz.com
Los Angeles branch. Support groups, information and other resources for adult women who experienced early mother loss.

Our House: www.ourhouse-grief.org
Based in Los Angeles, loving grief support for all ages.

SOME EXCEPTIONAL BOOKS

Motherless Daughters: The Legacy of Loss, by Hope Edelman
*Moving Beyond Grief: Lessons from Those Who Have
Lived Through Sorrow,* by Hope Edelman
On Death and Dying by Elizabeth Kubler-Ross M.D.
The Wheel of Life: A Memoir of Living and Dying,
by Elizabeth Kubler-Ross, Todd Gold
What's Heaven, by Maria Shriver / St. Martin's Press
*To Begin Again: The Journey Toward Comfort, Strength, and
Faith in Difficult Times,* by Naomi Levy

About the Authors

Gary Young's plays, mostly dealing with social issues, have been produced and performed at the Kennedy Center, Lincoln Center, the White House, the Smithsonian, and venues throughout the US and Europe. He has worked with Jean Kennedy Smith as a coordinator for the National Very Special Arts Festival, and has produced festivals and written successful grant proposals to fund programs for, by, and with disabled populations and the underprivileged. Funding agencies include the former HEW, National Endowment for the Arts, National Endowment for the Humanities, Mobil Oil, US Airlines, and several private foundations. His play, *Interruptions - A life, a death, pizza, dancing and Murphy's Law*, premiered at the Kennedy Center, and enjoyed a very successful West Coast premier in Los Angeles, June through September, 2000, at the Stella Adler Theatre in Hollywood.

Kathy Young has taught in the Colorado, Detroit, and the LA public schools, and has taught guitar and vocal music, and has written several children's books. She has worked with children in Afghanistan and Indonesia and she has traveled extensively around the world. After having children, she became a property supervisor, running four apartment buildings in addition to her own, a commercial complex, and an industrial complex. She was team mom for her children's sports teams, and continues to play an active role in her children's lives.

Kathy Young and **Gary Young** became co-leaders of some of the support groups that are mentioned in the book. Gary has had almost twenty years of experience with illness issues and death issues. Kathy has had over ten years of experience with illness and death issues.

They have recently discussed grief and recovery issues on *Leeza*, *The Home Show* (ABC), the *Dale Atkins Show* on Family TV, the *Marilyn Kagan Show* (Disney), and can be seen on *Between the Lines*, Barry Kibrick's acclaimed, in-depth, nationally syndicated review of major writers and their books. The TV movie, well, more about that later!

Order Form

Fax orders: Fax this form to (818) 222-5554

Phone orders: (818) 259-5553

Email: orders@calabashpress.com

Postal Orders: Calabash Press, P.O. Box 8728, Calabasas, Ca. 91372-8728

Books ordered may be returned for full refund within ten days.

Number of books @ $14.95:_____
Subtotal:_____
Tax:_____
Shipping:_____
Total Order: $_____

NOTE: Please add 8.25% **sales tax** for Ca. orders ($1.23 for one book)
Shipping: $2.00 for the first book, and $1.00 for each additional book
Please make checks/money orders out to **Calabash Press**.

Name:_____

Address_____

City_____State_____Zip_____-_____

Please send free information about:
☐ Other books   ☐ Speaking/Seminars

Payment: ☐ check   ☐ money order   ☐ credit card

☐ Visa   ☐ Mastercard   ☐ American Express   ☐ Discover

Card number:_____

Name on card:_____Exp. Date:___/___

Signature_____

The readers say:

"Such a moving and insightful aid! I particularly liked the truthful portrayal of both the male and female perspective."

"Your sensitivity, humor and clarity answered many of my questions, some of which I did not even know I had."

"I laughed a lot at the dating experiences. During the roughest time of my life, the book was my therapy and inspiration."

"I laughed and cried and realized that I am normal, and I am not alone! I could relate to both of your experiences."

"It's only been eight months, but I have seen a change in myself an din my life and I owe thanks to you for part of it."

"It's a great book, and once I started reading it, I couldn't put it down."

"It was particularly interesting to me to see an honest picture of a man crying. Your book will help many men who might feel that it is wrong to cry."